THE LAID BACK GUIDE TO INTERMITTENT FASTING

How I Lost Over 80 Pounds and Kept
It Off Eating Whatever I Wanted

Kayla Cox

CONTENTS

Title Page	1
Introduction	5
Chapter 1: My Journey	9
Chapter 2: Intermittent Fasting 101	22
Chapter 3: Intermittent Fasting Benefits	33
Chapter 4: Intermittent Fasting: Challenges	40
Chapter 5: Getting Started With Intermittent Fasting	49
Chapter 6: Going Off Plan	60
Chapter 7: My Daily Routine	65
Chapter 8: Cheat Day	68
Chapter 9: Intermittent Fasting and Exercise	75
Chapter 10: On The Importance of Tracking	81
Chapter 11: Intermittent Fasting And Periods	90
Chapter 12: Intermittent Fasting and Emotional Eating	94
Chapter 13: The Importance of Mindset	98
Chapter 14: How To Stay Motivated	104
Chapter 15: How To Maintain	109
Epilogue	112
About The Author	115
Books By This Author	117

This book is not intended as a substitute for the medical advice of physicians. It is for informational purposes only. The reader should regularly consult a physician in matters relating to his/her health and particularly with respect to any symptoms that may require diagnosis or medical attention.

INTRODUCTION

Become a possibilitarian. No matter how dark things seem to be or actually are, raise your sights and see possibilities -- always see them, for they're always there. -Norman Vincent Peale

What if you could eat whatever you wanted and still lose weight? It sounds too good to be true if you're a chronic dieter like I was. I always wished I could eat the same foods everyone else was enjoying and stay at a healthy weight. But that was never my reality. In order to lose weight, I always had to stop eating the foods I loved. Whenever I went back to eating those foods, I inevitably packed the pounds back on. The idea that I could actually lose weight while still eating my favorite foods seemed like a pipedream. Then I discovered intermittent fasting, and my lifelong weight loss dream came true.

I've hit the trifecta: I successfully lost over 80 pounds and haven't regained it, it felt easy and sustainable, and I have eaten whatever I wanted through the entire process. I went from being a chronic stress eater who had a horrible relationship with food, to a person who now trusts herself around all the foods, no matter how delicious. No foods are forbidden in my life. I feel free! I now eat to satiation, rather than misery on a regular basis. I am living proof that you don't have to practice intermittent fasting perfectly in order to have fantastic, sustainable results. In fact, I believe that the more laid back you are in your approach, the more success you will have.

I have adopted intermittent fasting as a lifestyle, and I only practice it 6 days a week. I also frequently take days off for special events, holidays, and vacations. I have found that intermittent fasting is a simple and easy way of life, and it offers a tremendous amount of flexibility. Unfortunately, that flexibility invites overcomplication, which then increases the level of difficulty unnecessarily. I am writing this book because I know from experience that you don't have to be super strict or make intermittent fasting difficult in order to reach a healthy weight. You can do it the easy way. It simply takes patience and persistence over time. I want you to know that if I can do it, anyone can. I am not special. In fact, I'm probably a lot like you.

A little backstory on me: I've ridden the weight loss roller coaster my entire life. From age 6 until 32, I always felt like I was either overweight and unhappy about it, on a diet and miserable, or in the process of gaining the weight back. And every time I gained the weight back, it got a little bit harder to get the motivation to try to lose the weight again. By the time I had my third baby, I felt like I was fighting a losing battle. I tried very hard to learn how to be happy about being overweight, but I just couldn't do it.

The Photo That Started It All

One day in early 2014, I got a notification on Facebook that I'd been tagged in some photos from my brother-in-law's 30th birthday party. I happily tapped on the notification, fully expecting to see cute photos of my kids. Although my youngest was almost two, I still hadn't lost the baby weight, and routinely dodged the camera at all costs. As I scrolled through the pictures, I realized to my horror that my camera radar hadn't been working at all that day. My face was red hot and I was blinking back tears. There were lots of photos of me, and from every unflattering angle. I hardly recognized myself. I was mortified when I realized how much in denial I had been about my weight. I locked myself in the bathroom. I sat down on the floor and let my tears flow for as long as they would come. And then I got angry. Angry at Facebook for having that stupid tagging feature. Angry at the person who'd taken the photos. Angry at the smartphone manufacturers for making cameras omnipresent in our lives. And then I finally got angry with the person truly responsible for my plight: me. I started to pray. I felt the anger start to dissipate. I decided to pick myself up, and dust myself off. From that point on, I was determined to find a way to get the weight off once and for all.

I wish I could tell you that the very next day, I heard about intermittent fasting, implemented it perfectly, and got down to my ideal weight quickly and with no effort at all. In reality, it was a messy journey, with tons of failure, self-doubt, and inconsistency. I lost some weight, almost drove myself crazy obsessing over calories and macros, plateaued for months, came close to giving up, and then finally found what worked for me. As it turns out, my main mistake in the beginning was making things more complicated than they needed to be.

My Hope

I vividly remember how frustrated I felt in 2014. Even though I was severely overweight, I could not bear the thought of going on yet another diet. I hate the word *diet*. It immediately brings to my mind the disgusting, chunky "chocolate" protein shakes I would gulp down in my teenage years when I was trying to get down to a healthy weight. No diet had ever worked for me over the long term. I wanted so badly to find a way to lose weight and maintain it easily for the rest of my life. I wanted to be able to eat regular food, with no complicated rules or calculations necessary. I knew that would be the only sustainable path for me. I found that path with intermittent fasting.

I know first-hand the dread you feel when you are losing weight, but deep down you know you'll eventually go back to eating all the delicious foods you really love. I want you to know that you can continue to eat all the foods you love. My experience has taught me that you don't have to say goodbye to cheesecake or chocolate. You do not have to count calories. You do not even have to limit carbs. Intermittent fasting is the only way of eating that I've been able to stick to consistently for years, with what feels like very little effort, all while feeling fantastic and eating whatever foods I'm craving. While successful weight loss and maintenance has been an amazing result, I've also found other major benefits. Intermittent fasting gives me loads of energy, helped me stop stress eating, improved my relationship with food in general, increased my productivity and focus, and has improved my quality of life overall.

My hope is that I can make the concept of intermittent fasting simple and easy for you, too. I hope you can learn from my mistakes. It took me two years of searching, researching and experimenting before I found and implemented intermittent fasting successfully. I'll share my successes and failures, and give you tips on how to make it easier on yourself, based on what I've learned. I'll show you exactly how I do intermittent fasting, including how I track my progress and the mindset shifts that have happened, which have been crucial to my long-term results.

Let's also touch briefly on what this book is *not*. It's not medical advice. I'm not a doctor, and you should discuss all diet and exercise decisions with your healthcare provider. I'm not a psychologist, and this is not mental health advice. If you have psychological issues, please seek out professional help immediately. There is no shame in reaching out for help. This book is also not nutrition advice. I'm still a major work in progress in this department. This is not even a book about the *right* way to do intermittent fasting. My personal belief is there is no one right way. Furthermore, I believe that intermittent fasting is not for everyone. What follows is simply the way that worked for me. I hope this book will serve as a launching off point for you. I hope you customize your own plan to your needs, your life, and your goals. I have found it quite empowering to chart my own course and make my own rules, and I hope you will, too.

CHAPTER 1: MY JOURNEY

If you could kick the person in the pants responsible for most of your trouble, you wouldn't sit for a month. -Theodore Roosevelt

I think a quick overview of my journey will be helpful, though feel free to skip ahead to the next chapter if you're more interested in the ins and outs of intermittent fasting.

2014

After my come to Jesus moment in my bathroom in 2014, I spent the rest of the year focused on trying to figure out what I could try to solve my weight problem, but I didn't take much action. I tried to move more, eat better, and I started taking progress photos. Even though I wasn't showing any progress, the photos served as a reality check, a weekly reminder of where I was. If anything, I'd no longer be surprised by how I looked in pictures. I started reading a lot of self-help books, which ended up being crucial to my long term success. I had spurts of being more active. For several months I jogged three miles a day. But when I didn't notice any real results, I gave up. Ultimately I balked at the idea of changing what foods I was eating. When I looked at my pattern of weight loss and weight gain, I saw that while I could easily get rid of certain foods in the short term, I eventually went back to eating them when I got the weight off. My goal was to find some way of eating which allowed me to eat any kinds of food I wanted. It seemed like wishful thinking. But I kept searching on the Internet, and as luck would have it, in late 2014, I finally stumbled across intermittent fasting.

You would hope that's when everything fell into place for me, but that's just not how it happened. Intermittent fasting couldn't be simpler. You don't eat for a certain amount of time each day. It really is that straightforward. But as a human, I have a tendency to overcomplicate things. I experience analysis paralysis. In my case it looks like this: I hear about a diet or exercise regimen. I then proceed to bury myself in researching it, how to do it perfectly, and all the possible risks and benefits, ad nauseam. Meanwhile, I don't actually *try* the thing. I just keep researching and delaying action, sometimes indefinitely. On December 7, 2014, I started dabbling with intermittent fasting. It was so different from every other piece of weight loss wisdom out there that it made me hesitant to go ahead fullsteam. Would skipping meals put my body in starvation mode? Would I just binge on food if I waited longer between meals? But still, the idea of it fascinated me, so I just kind of played with it. I found it rather easy. I also found I felt good while I was doing it. But I was terrified I'd mess up my hormones if I did this long term or if my fasts were too long, which kept me from being consistent.

2015

By February 2015, I was frustrated that the progress photos weren't showing any real progress, so I took my sister-in-law up on her offer to try out the gym she was going to. I felt completely out of place as I walked through the locker room. I had flashbacks of having to change out for gym class in middle school, an already embarrassing ritual made worse by my "fluffiness" as my gym teacher once referred to it. And to top it all off, there in the corner loomed my arch-nemesis: the scale. I had refused to weigh myself since the birth of my third child. I timidly entered the women's only gym area. I walked around, trying to pretend like I knew what I was doing.

I finally crawled onto the elliptical machine and watched on in envy as women with tiny waists and chiseled abs bounced confidently out of the protection of our women's cave into the terrifying mixed use area with bodybuilders and powerlifters galore. The designers of the gym, for what I can only assume were sadistic reasons, lined the walls of the women's gym with mirrors. I was forced to stare at myself as I exercised, red-faced and jiggly all over. I was angry. I started punishing myself on that machine for not making any noticeable progress on my weight problem. A battle was going on inside my head. *I am so overweight! Look at how my belly is flopping up and down. Wait! Am I being overly critical? Maybe I'm not that overweight! I bet I don't weigh as much as I think I do. What if I weigh more?*

After killing myself on the elliptical for several minutes, my curiosity got the better of me. I needed to find out how much I actually weighed. Ironically, in 2014 I'd chosen not to weigh myself for fear of being a slave to the scale. But slave I was, despite not knowing. I constantly worried and wondered how much I weighed, and if I was losing any weight. But since I refused to weigh, I had no idea if any of my efforts were working. I finally stepped off the machine, went back into the locker room, and approached my foe. Whether my heart felt like it was beating out of my chest because of the cardio, or because of my sheer terror, I'll never know. I finally got my courage up and looked my fear in the face. I expected to see 185 staring back at me. Instead, I saw 222, which at 5'6" put me firmly in the obese category according to the Body Mass Index (BMI).

This was a major turning point in my journey. Up until that point, I had been in a lot of denial about where I was, despite taking the weekly progress photos. Having the cold, hard facts made me get serious about taking action. I had a renewed resolve to get rid of my weight problems once and for all. Intermittent fasting was the only eating plan that had interested me, so I decided to commit to it. The idea that I just needed to control *when* I ate, not *what* I ate, appealed to me. It sounded sustainable. I started out with very short fasting windows and worked my way up to longer fasts. I had read an article somewhere, thanks to my copious research, that said women should not consistently fast more than 14 hours each day, and I tried to follow that. I went to the gym every single day, did crossfit 3 days a week, and eventually started powerlifting. My idea was to change my eating gradually, but work out as hard as I could.

I had some initial success. Intermittent fasting felt easy, and I really got into powerlifting. The weight was coming down gradually. I slowly gained confidence, and eventually I was out there lifting heavy weights with all the other powerlifters. In mid-April I decided to start logging all of my food intake in the hopes my weight loss would speed up. At that point I had lost about a pound a week on average. At first, I didn't mind logging my food. Over time, however, I began to resent it. I was surrounded by people who were maintaining a perfectly healthy weight, and I noticed none of them were getting on their phones and inputting every bite of food they ate. I would go to Chick-Fil-A and order my favorite, the chicken strips. If I ordered the 3 count, it was only 330 calories. But then, what are chicken strips without the sauce? And that's when I began to utterly loathe the process of food tracking. Every delicious sauce packet was 140 calories. That's okay, I told myself. I'll just have one. I'd sparingly use my sauce packet, wiping it absolutely clean with the last of the strips. But instead of feeling proud of myself at the end of the meal, I felt deprived. I tried to convince myself that this was just my reality. Other people could eat what they like and not track their food, but I was just different. My weight loss journey started to feel more difficult, but still I pressed on.

And then I hit another snag. At the end of June I injured my back due to deadlifting with poor form. This stressed me out because I wasn't able to work out as aggressively. I kept going to the gym, trying to heal and keep active. By the end of July I was down a total of 20 pounds, to a seven day average weight of 202. That was an average loss of a pound a week. And do you know how I felt? Like a big fat failure. I was shocked that logging my food wasn't making the progress faster. My real goal in 2015 was to lose 5 pounds a week and be done with this weight loss nonsense within a few months. Instead of feeling proud of how much progress I had made, I was frustrated that I wasn't done yet, and still had so far to go. It had been five months of hard work, and I wasn't out of the 200s yet. I told myself I just needed to work harder.

And this is where I made a huge mistake. I started getting obsessed with the food I was eating. For the next several months, I started counting my calories and figuring out my macros. I spent lots of my precious time trying to find the exact match of what I was eating in the Fitbit food database. It wasn't enough for me to select "black bean burger" from the list. I calculated all the calories based on the exact recipe I had used, including exact measurements of the condiments. Each meal started to become a real pain in the butt. And do you know what all that stress and effort got me? A plateau. A big, fat, weight loss plateau. I kept telling myself to keep at it, that the plateau would eventually break, and that I just needed to be even more exact with the food tracking I was doing. I started weighing and measuring all of my food.

I remember one night in particular. We were having tacos. I love my tacos with copious toppings, especially cheese. As it turns out, an actual serving of shredded cheese is ¼ of a cup. When I dug that sad little ¼ cup of cheese out of the bag with my measuring cup, and then sprinkled it on my tacos, I died a little inside. I looked around the table. My husband, who's been a skinny guy his entire life, was happily piling cheese and sour cream on his taco with abandon. My kids were eating as many tacos as they wanted, perfectly clueless as to macros, calories, and suggested serving sizes. And yet I, despite all my efforts, was the only overweight one at the table. I desperately wanted their reality to be my reality. I had had it! If they didn't have to count calories, neither did I! On

October 8, 2015, I decided to stop counting calories, once and for all. I told myself I was going to simply try to eat intuitively. I would stop eating when I felt full. I still experimented with intermittent fasting, and I was doing 12-13 hour fasts during this time. I was still paranoid that prolonged intermittent fasting would mess up my hormones or my metabolism, so I didn't practice it consistently.

My seven day average weight hovered right above 200 from July 2015 on through December of that year. During that plateau, my eating and exercise was all over the map. I'd quit intermittent fasting, because I was afraid that it was causing my metabolism to slow down. But then my weight would start to trend up, and so I'd go back to it. I'd set step goals and reach them for a while, and then quit walking because it didn't seem hard enough. I started to wonder whether I was being realistic in my plan to not go on another diet. A lot of my friends were having success with keto and paleo, but I knew in my heart of hearts I would not be able to stick to any kind of diet like that over the long term.

2016

By January 2016, I was at the point of giving up. My weight continued to hover at a seven day average of 205. Up to this point I was afraid to do anything consistently longer than a 14 hour fast on a regular basis for fear it would mess up my hormones. I decided that remaining overweight was a bigger risk. I decided to start pushing my fasting window out further, but I didn't really have a true plan. I had been reading many personal development books since 2014, but I had refused to read any diet books during this time. Over my lifetime, I had tried plenty of diets, and they'd never stuck. Reading yet another diet book felt like I was admitting failure, but I was desperate.

I had been a big fan of Tim Ferriss since 2014 when I read his book *The 4 Hour Work Week*. I was drawn to his unique perspective on various topics. I knew he'd written a book called *The 4 Hour Body* and I figured it was worth a shot. In the book he recommends the slow carb diet. I tried it for about two days before I realized that eliminating "white carbs" like potatoes and rice simply wasn't sustainable for my life. I love bread, pasta, and pretty much every carb out there, and I knew myself well enough to know they'd always be a part of my life. Ferriss also mentioned Seth Roberts, who had created his own weight loss method called the Shangri-La diet. I tried it too, again for about two days, before I realized that drinking two tablespoons of sugar water twice a day wasn't going to be sustainable for me either. Despite that, I gleaned a very important concept from this book: I realized that I could simply make up my own plan.

My Plan

It might sound silly, but the thought had never occurred to me. I suppose I thought all the experts out there were the only ones who had permission to create eating plans. While I didn't follow Ferriss' diet plan, I did glean mindset advice and a few hacks from his book. It was the first time I had considered the idea of simply thinking of a weight loss plan as an experiment. Because of my shift in mindset, I decided to sit down and write out my own plan for an experiment. One important trick I learned from Ferriss was to ask the question, "What would this look like if it were easy?" I decided weight loss would be easy if I could:
- Eat whatever I wanted
- Drink coffee whenever I wanted
- Have a cheat day every Sunday (another tip from Ferriss)
- Walk at a slow pace as my exercise

I knew at this point that to lose weight, I needed to have some sort of boundary with food. By this time I had found that intermittent fasting in general felt easy to me. I was very good with time boundaries with food. I decided to run this as a 6 week experiment. To sum up, my plan was this:

- Intermittent fasting 6 days a week
    - Eat whatever I want during the eating window
        - Eat however much I want
        - No counting calories
        - No limiting carbs
    - Coffee with half and half whenever I wanted it during the fasting window
- Cheat day on Sunday
- Walk 6 miles a day

Quite frankly, I expected this experiment to completely blow up in my face. It seemed too easy. Too good to be true. I thought I would gain 5 or 6 pounds, but in reality I dropped 7 pounds. A little more than a pound a week! With what felt like no effort! After such a long plateau, I was in disbelief. At that point, I gave myself permission to run this as an experiment for the rest of the year. I knew that if I could keep up the pound a week weight loss, my weight would be near a normal BMI by the holidays.

Because it felt so easy, I stuck to this plan consistently and I had consistent results. In January my fasts were about 16 hours long. I gradually pushed out my fasting window as I felt comfortable, and by April I started simply eating one meal a day (OMAD). By November 2016, I was down to a seven day average weight of 157. With the holidays upon me, I decided to try to maintain my weight loss for a while. I didn't know how easy or hard it would be.

November 2016-September 2017

As it turns out, maintenance was almost effortless. This felt too good to be true. I tested out variations of intermittent fasting to see what would keep the weight off, and I found I could be very flexible with my eating and still stay within 5 pounds of my lowest weight. Surprisingly, I found that I felt the best when I continued to do some form of intermittent fasting. I found that my preferred way to maintain was to continue to walk 6 miles a day, have supper as my first meal, and then enjoy evening snacks with my husband.

September 2017 - Present

By September of 2017, I was thoroughly convinced of the sustainability of intermittent fasting. When I first began, I wasn't sure how long I could stick with this way of eating. But when I was in maintenance mode I realized how easy and sustainable it was, and how I truly preferred intermittent fasting as a way of life. I decided to start a Youtube channel in order to tell others about how I found weight loss success with intermittent fasting and walking. Since I was still a few pounds overweight according to my BMI, I decided it was time to lose a bit more. I went back to my original plan, and as of this writing I'm down to a seven day average of 140, for a total weight loss of 82 pounds.

Timeline Analysis

Why did I have weight loss success in 2016, but not so much in 2015? Certainly if you look at 2015, I was working out much harder, and doing more difficult things, food-wise. The following year I did almost the complete opposite and I lost three times as much weight. For me, it comes down to three important things: proper mindset, long-term consistency, and easiness.

Mindset Shifts

In 2015 I was in a huge rush. I wanted to drop major weight fast and be done with my weight loss within a few months. A pound a week of loss felt like failure. I had it in my head that slow results weren't good. I thought it meant I wasn't trying hard enough. I ended up making it harder and harder on myself, which led to inconsistency. Luckily, my mindset started to change thanks to the self-improvement books I was reading.

By 2016, thanks to Darren Hardy's book *The Compound Effect*, I understood the power of small, sustainable changes over time. Instead of being in a hurry, I became patient. I finally gave myself permission for this to take a long time. Instead of aiming for losing five pounds a week, my goal was one pound a week. I realized that one pound a week meant 52 pounds a year. I even accepted the idea of losing a half a pound a week, if necessary. If it took me two years to get down to a good weight, so be it. It took me years to pack on the pounds, after all. I was finally willing to sacrifice speed for sustainability.

The experimental mindset I gleaned from Tim Ferriss was tremendously important. It helped me to try things I wouldn't have otherwise felt brave enough to do. It also helped me emotionally to start thinking like a scientist. Instead of thinking of myself as a failure, I could step outside the situation and look at it as the subject (me) didn't do well with the experiment. Before beginning to think like this, my tendency was to get very emotional about my weight. Any weight gains or fluctuations would ruin my day. When I switched to an experimental mindset, I could be curious instead of emotional.

I was able to unemotionally look at the data I was collecting and see that the plan was working. This made my daily weigh-ins less stressful as well. I began to look at each weigh-in as a data point that would give me insight, which kept me weighing consistently. This in turn lessened my fear of weighing, until it became another mundane task, much like brushing my teeth. This constant stream of data showed me how various foods affected my weight, and whether these changes were permanent or transient. A hugely important thing I've learned is that while many foods will cause a temporary rise in weight, none of them cause me permanent weight gain. This led to the realization that I could still eat every single kind of food, as long as I had some sort of boundaries with them. Intermittent fasting provided the time boundary I needed.

Consistency

When I formed my plan, I committed to it fully for six weeks. The agreement with myself was six weeks was enough time to see how I was doing with the plan, and to see some results. At the end of six weeks, I'd lost a little over 7 pounds. I considered this a major success, because it felt so completely easy. I was eating large portions, eating whatever foods I wanted, and I wasn't measuring, tracking, or doing any calculations. I figured that I could commit to staying consistent on such an easy plan, especially if I could continue to have results like that.

My consistency during 2016 was spectacular. I don't believe I skipped a single day of walking 6 miles, and my eating plan stayed very consistent as well, though I did have to learn how to go off plan when necessary. My results reflect that consistency. Although my weight didn't go down every single day, overall it was a fairly consistent downward trend with no long plateaus. My plan was very simple, and I believe this contributed to my ability to be very consistent. It didn't require any complex calculations or special foods. But more important than its simplicity was how easy it felt.

Easiness

The plan feeling easy was crucial to my success. The weight loss journey is long. Willpower is a limited resource, as I found out the hard way with every single diet plan I ever tried. I can resist chocolate cake for months if necessary, but eventually my willpower runs out. Eventually I will go back to eating the chocolate cake. I wanted this weight loss plan to feel easy. I literally wanted to have my cake and eat it too. And so that's how I formed this plan. All the foods were allowed. The only thing that wasn't allowed was guilt. I believe the reason I was able to give myself permission to create such an easy plan was because I saw it as an experiment. There is something very freeing about calling something an experiment. You can try something that seems silly or unconventional. I have been able to apply this to other areas of my life as well, and it's led to some incredible adventures, such as our family's current experiment in full-time RVing across America.

Unexpected Results

When I formed this plan, I had serious doubts that it would work. In fact, I figured my results would be that I would gain weight. When I look at the results I had in 2016, I'm reminded of another tactic I learned from Tim Ferriss: it is helpful to ask yourself sometimes, *what if I did the opposite*? In the past with weight loss, I tried to make it as hard on myself as possible. I did the hardest workouts, and demanded of myself that I stick to the diet 100% perfectly. The plan I formed in 2016 was almost the opposite of that.

My weekly cheat day made it so that I was never more than a B + student of intermittent fasting. I was only intermittent fasting 6 days a week, or 85% of the time, so it prevented me from ever thinking I was being perfect. This plan felt almost too easy. I was allowing myself all the delicious food I used to think I really shouldn't allow myself to eat. My "workout" was just a slow six mile walk. And even that wasn't a bona fide workout. I counted every step I got during the normal course of my day. Sometimes I would just do my steps in 10 or 15 minute chunks and then sit down and rest. It was all about whatever felt easiest. It was almost the anti-diet. And yet, by the end of 2016 I had dropped my weight to 157.

Chapter Notes

- My weight loss journey had 3 major turning points:
    - The day I said "I've had enough" (March 24, 2014)
    - The day I weighed myself (February 20, 2015)
    - The day that I created my own plan (January 6, 2016)
- Lessons I learned on my journey
    - I found the best plan when I asked myself what plan would be **easy** to stick to.
    - It was freeing to create a plan, commit to it and run it as a six week experiment.
    - It was best to focus on consistency rather than speed of weight loss.
    - It was reasonable to set a goal of 1 pound of weight loss per week on average.
    - It was best to focus on the big picture. I had the most success when I started to think in terms of months and years instead of days and even weeks.
    - Err on the side of making the plan too easy.
    - Aim for being a B+ student. It's freeing.
    - There is value in asking yourself, "What if I did the opposite?"

CHAPTER 2: INTERMITTENT FASTING 101

Start the practice of self-control with some penance; begin with fasting. -Mahavira

So what is intermittent fasting, anyway? It's simply not eating for a certain portion of the day. Your time is divided into the fasting window and the eating window. The fasting window is the period of time in which you do not eat. The eating window is the period of time in which you eat. Generally intermittent fasting refers to fasts of 24 hours or less, whereas extended fasting covers fasts for longer than that. This book will only discuss intermittent fasting, as I have no experience yet with extended fasting. The fasting window and the eating window add up to 24 hours. Some examples of the written format describing what kind of intermittent fasting you're doing looks like this:
- 16:8 means your fasting window is 16 hours long, and your eating window is 8 hours long
- 20:4 means your fasting window is 20 hours long, and your eating window is 4 hours long

In real life a 16:8 could look like this:
- Between the hours of 9 pm and 1 pm you do not eat (16 hours of fasting)
- Between the hours of 1 pm and 9 pm you eat (8 hours of eating)

You pick the time you want your windows to be, and the length you want them to be. An 8 hour eating window does not mean you eat non-stop during the entire 8 hours. It simply means you only eat food during the 8 hour period. You might eat 2 meals during that time, or 2 meals and snacks, or all snacks, depending on what you prefer. You may find that you are ready for a big meal when your eating window opens, and then that big meal keeps you full until your next meal near the end of your window.

How Does Intermittent Fasting Work?

If you want to know all the ins and outs of the science behind intermittent fasting, I highly recommend you go check out Dr. Jason Fung, a kidney specialist who is an amazing advocate for the health benefits of fasting. He has written several books and has a website with extensive research about the science behind intermittent fasting.

As you will recall, I am not a medical doctor, a scientist, nor a nutritionist, but I can offer a quick and dirty explanation of intermittent fasting. Basically, your body needs energy in order to function. It can either get that energy from the food that you eat, or the fat that you've stored. When you are overweight, you have plenty of fat stored. Your body first uses the food you've eaten most recently for energy, because it's more readily available. When you have longer blocks of time of not eating, your body enters the fasted state. Your body must start burning through the stored fat in order to continue functioning. When your body burns stored fat, you lose weight.

Fasting Window Rules

What can you have during the fasting window? Technically, you simply shouldn't eat anything. The goal is to get into and remain in a fasted state, and this is not something that is well defined in science. It's probably more accurate to think of the fasted state and the fed state as two ends of a spectrum. Generally your body is in a fasted state 12 hours after your last food was eaten. If you decide to eat 50 calories worth of an apple 12 hours after your last meal, will it kick you out of the fasted state? Probably not. It's probably more accurate to say you're in a less fasted state until you can burn through those calories, which is generally a small window of time. Unfortunately, at this point not a lot of scientific studies have been done regarding intermittent fasting. We find ourselves getting into a gray area. This is where I find experimentation is exceedingly helpful.

What about coffee with cream and sugar? What about tea? Artificial sweeteners? Gum? Mints? Protein shakes? This is where you're going to start getting ten different answers if you ask ten different intermittent fasters. I take the most laid back approach. I say experiment with it, and see what works for you. I've always allowed myself whatever I felt like I needed in the window. I regularly had mints, gum, and coffee with cream and sugar during my fasting window in the beginning. I say, if it will get you through the fasting window without actually eating, try it. Be super consistent with it, and record your results. There is no intermittent fasting police that will come and get you if you have a coffee with half and half and sugar in your fasting window. I speak from experience.

Making The Fasting Window Easier

Most people find intermittent fasting at least somewhat challenging in the beginning. The idea of not eating the instant I felt any hunger was almost scary to me. I was terrified that my metabolism would slow down and it would be impossible to lose weight. As the weight started to come off, I started to realize my fears had been unfounded. With time, I realized that I was going to be okay if I waited a bit to eat. Intermittent fasting gets easier as time goes on. And fortunately, I found many ways to make the fasting window easier.

Stay Busy

When you are fasting, do not sit around and think about food. Stay busy. **This is probably the most important tip for successful fasting, period.** I used the fasting window to my advantage. I discovered I had a lot more time available to me than I previously realized, and I used that time to be super productive. I cleaned house, got my six miles of walking in, learned a second language (American Sign Language), learned how to build Android apps, read books, started drawing again, played with my kids, and just got stuff done in general. I found that filling up my life this way also made me a happier person. If you find you are bored during the fasting window, actively find some new hobbies and interests, or perhaps go volunteer out in your community. Just find a way to stay busy!

Coffee

Coffee was a life-saver for me as I pushed out my fasting window. Having coffee with half and half (or sometimes heavy cream) always took the edge off my hunger and helped me stick to the fasting window. It also served another purpose. When you're fasting, you're usually missing out on a meal or two with your spouse/significant other. This can make one or both of you feel like you're missing out on time together that you used to enjoy. Having coffee together helped my husband and I reconnect throughout the day, and solved that issue for us.

Beverage Variety

Of course, you can always have as much water as you want throughout your fasting window. And it can also help keep you feeling full. However, if you're anything like me, you'll get bored with plain water. Sugar during the fasting window is supposedly a no-no, so over time I trained myself to like unsweetened beverages by slowly weaning myself off of sugar in my drinks in 2015. To give you an idea of how sweet I liked my drinks in the beginning, I used to make my sweet tea with 1.5 cups of sugar in one gallon of tea and my coffee with one tablespoon of sugar in each mugful. To learn to like unsweetened drinks, I cut the sugar by small increments, and learned to enjoy it that way before cutting more. Now I truly enjoy coffee with cream and no sugar, and unsweetened tea. And even better, fasting became easier when I eliminated the sugar from my drinks.

I have also found that unsweetened flavored sodas are quite a treat. I do not enjoy artificial sweeteners, so Diet Cokes are out for me. Drinks like La Croix and Bubly, which do not have any sweeteners at all taste wonderful to me now. Be forewarned: if you currently love sweet soda, you will probably hate the taste of unsweetened soda. I first had to train myself to enjoy unsweetened beverages, and only then did I begin to enjoy these drinks. I love a nice, refreshing, bubbly beverage, and these really hit the spot.

Stay Consistent
The more consistent you can be with keeping your fasting window at the same length and time each day, the easier it will feel. Don't try to recalculate your window based on what time you ate your last food each day. This will save you a lot of stress and confusion. It will also make it feel easier, because your body will get used to not eating during your fasting window. If you're constantly changing your window, you're going to feel more hunger, period.

Eating Window Rules

My rule is, I eat whatever I want and however much I want during my eating window. I do not have a meal plan. The idea of giving myself complete and total freedom, no guilty feelings allowed, was quite scary at first. I didn't think I could be trusted with food. But I told myself no guilty feelings were allowed. As long as I was sticking to my eating window, I was allowed any kind of food I wanted. It didn't matter how delicious, or rich, or fattening. Desserts? Totally allowed! Pasta? Yes, please! Chocolate? However much you want!

Ad Libitum Eating

I figured I'd binge on all these foods, now that they were all allowed. But a funny thing happened. When all the foods were allowed, the "bad foods" kind of lost their luster, and I ended up eating them less often. Previous to this, I was the type of person who always felt that I was being bad if I ate certain foods, like chocolate chip cookies. This would lead to a crazy back and forth in my head while I was eating the aforementioned cookies. I would end up overindulging, because of all the inner turmoil and stress. I would eat until I was miserable. It was almost rebellion. *You think I shouldn't be allowed chocolate chip cookies? I'll show you!*

But now that I was allowing myself to eat whatever I wanted, chocolate chip cookies included, no guilty feelings allowed, I ate the cookies, but without the emotional baggage. I was following my plan. This wasn't cheating. Chocolate chip cookies were now just chocolate chip cookies. Delicious? Yes. Heavenly? Yes. But laden with guilt and stress? No. I found I could eat decadent chocolate cake that I previously couldn't control myself around. I started to tell myself I could have as many pieces as I wanted. And generally, I found that I actually wanted just one. And I stopped there. Not because I was trying to be good, but rather because one piece was how much I actually wanted to eat. Do I sometimes eat more than one piece of chocolate cake? Sure! Do I beat myself up if I have more? Nope! Because I'm following my plan, and my rules.

The goal with ad libitum eating is not to stuff yourself until you're absolutely miserable. Instead, it's a learning process of figuring out:
- Which foods you enjoy
- Which foods you do not enjoy
- Which foods you feel best eating
- How much of the food you should eat to feel completely full
- How much food will make you uncomfortably full

Eating to misery is the opposite of ad libitum. Ad libitum is Latin for at one's pleasure. Eating to misery is not pleasurable. It took me a while to figure out the sweet spot. Sometimes I would overdo it on a food and feel uncomfortably full. Other times I wouldn't eat quite enough of the thing and found that I would crave it more. The main thing that helped me was to be kind to myself. I refused to beat myself up if I messed up, which helped me to continually improve.

Calories

Do you need to count calories when you're intermittent fasting? I do not. In 2015 when I started counting calories, I quickly became obsessed with the calorie count of everything. I found the overall stress and effort it took did not make the weight loss any faster for me. Am I saying counting calories doesn't work? Absolutely not. Tons of people have great success with it. It's just that it drove me crazy. I made a personal decision in 2015 to never count calories again, and I've stuck to it.

Carbs

Do you have to limit carbs? I do not. If anything, I tend to eat higher carb. Carbs are cheap, and we're a family of five on a budget. I have found that I function and feel the best when I'm getting plenty of carbs. And I'm not just talking kale and brussel sprouts. I'm talking white rice, beans, white bread, and regular ol' semolina pasta. I also eat dessert whenever I take a notion, which is usually about once a week. I have found that for me personally, I feel the best throughout the day if I have eaten plenty of carbs, protein, and fat at my meal. If I try to eat one to the exclusion of all others, I don't have the best energy levels. This is purely anecdotal. I think you should experiment with your own way of eating and see how you feel best. I've spoken with people who thrive on both ends of the spectrum, from carnivore to vegan.

Portions

When I set up my plan, I thought about portions. I decided that my rule would be, I'll eat however much I want. I like big portions, and I knew that for me, telling myself to eat small portions would just lead to me feeling deprived, and this plan would feel hard. My general idea was to not be in misery, either from eating too little and feeling hungry during my fasting window, or from eating too much and feeling overfull after my meal. I love large portions, and I allowed myself to keep them on this plan.

My appetite fluctuates during the month, and therefore so do my portions. During certain times, I require less food, and at other times, I need more. I have learned to listen to my body and to obey my appetite. I do not freak out or feel guilty when I eat more servings than I normally do. I figure hormonal fluctuations are the cause behind it.

Alcohol
I have found that I can drink wine with my meal and it won't affect my weight loss. I have a glass whenever I like. I don't drink more than two glasses in general, because my tolerance for alcohol is rather low. I have noticed that if I drink a glass of wine a few hours after my meal, I'll feel hunger during my fasting window the next day, and occasionally some nausea. It hasn't affected my weight loss, only the difficulty of the fasting window. I don't regularly drink liquor, but I have had an occasional drink, and again, it's never affected my weight loss. I encourage you to do your own experiments and see what works for you.

Restaurants
When forming my plan, I knew eating at restaurants would be at least a weekly thing with my family. We go to a restaurant or get take out at least once, but sometimes twice a week. I have no special rules about trying to limit how often we go to restaurants, nor what I eat when I am there. I simply order and eat whatever I want, and however much I want. Be forewarned, you'll probably notice a temporary increase in water weight after eating takeout,

especially Mexican and Chinese. I've found the extra weight goes away in a couple of days, and my weight continues to trend downward in the right direction over time, but it can be a tough thing to wait out the first few times it happens.

Omad (One Meal A Day)

One meal a day, or OMAD as it will be referred to for the remainder of this book, is my preferred way to practice intermittent fasting. It's truly as simple as it sounds: you eat once a day. When I refer to OMAD I am referring to literally eating one meal per day. I have found OMAD to be the simplest way to do intermittent fasting. You sit down and eat your one meal each day. When you stand up from the table, you begin your fasting again, and do not eat until your one meal the next day.

I have found several benefits to OMAD specifically. I don't have to think about windows, which simplifies my life. I tend to be the type of person who loses track of what time, and even what day it is. Heck, sometimes I forget what month we're in. It also saves a lot of time. I'm only preparing, eating, and cleaning up a single meal. I find I'm very productive during the day, because I only need to think about eating once. I never realized how much of my time was spent standing in the kitchen, trying to figure out what to eat, until I started practicing OMAD.

Does OMAD offer faster weight loss than a 16:8? That was my window in January 2016, when I formed my plan. I was losing about a pound a week at that time. Would my weight loss have slowed, or even stopped if I had simply stayed on a 16:8 over time? I do not know. I pushed my window out further, as it felt easy, because I figured I'd lose quicker, but that didn't happen. I reached OMAD accidentally, and found that I loved that style of eating, so I stuck with it. But over time my weight loss on OMAD was also about a pound a week on average. My general thought is, you should stick with a way of intermittent fasting that provides you with steady results and that you can be very consistent with. I don't believe OMAD is the holy grail of weight loss. It's quite possible I would have had the same results if I had just stuck to a 16:8. I simply prefer OMAD as a way of life.

2Mad (Two Meals A Day)

I'd be remiss if I didn't mention 2MAD, which is simply eating two meals a day. Some people keep the two meals at a consistent time, and others don't. The basic idea is two meals, and no snacks. I've never tried this plan, so I cannot comment on it.

Is Intermittent Fasting Healthy?

The main concern I had when I started intermittent fasting was that it seemed to go completely against the grain of generally accepted weight loss guidelines. Instead of breakfast being sacred, it was okay to skip it. Instead of eating five times a day, you might eat only once or twice a day. I worried that I would become nutrient deficient. Would I be starving myself? I'm not a nutritionist, or a doctor. I urge you to talk over all those things with your healthcare professional and draw your own conclusions. I researched the risks and benefits of intermittent fasting thoroughly before deciding to try it. I also armed myself with the knowledge of the symptoms of nutrient deficiency, just in case. For what it's worth, I've never suffered any symptoms of nutrient deficiency or starvation, even after practicing intermittent fasting for years.

My general philosophy has been to focus on getting the weight off first, before I try to perfect my food intake, as far as what I eat. Unfortunately, the more I research it, the more I'm confused. Some people emphasize how important getting lots of fruits and veggies are, which seems perfectly reasonable. But then I'll find out that other people are trumpeting the benefits of a strict carnivore diet, with admittedly impressive results. At this point,

I subscribe to Mark Twain's maxim: "Part of the secret of success in life is to eat what you like and let the food fight it out inside." I simply do not stress over what to eat, and instead pay attention to how I'm feeling. Overall, I have found that I have never felt better than when I am eating once a day and eating a wide variety of foods. I urge you to find the balance that works for you.

Chapter Notes

- Intermittent fasting means you do not eat for a certain period of time each day
- You do not eat during your fasting window
- You eat during your eating window
- To make the fasting window easier:
    - Stay busy
    - Drink coffee
    - Get some beverage variety in your life
    - Keep your fasting window at the same time each day
- My eating window rules
    - Eat whatever I want, no guilt allowed
    - No counting calories
    - No restricting carbs or portions
    - I drink alcohol when I take a notion (generally 1 glass of wine at dinner)
    - I eat at restaurants/get take out at least once a week, and many times twice.
- OMAD means One Meal A Day
    - I prefer OMAD because of the simplicity

CHAPTER 3: INTERMITTENT FASTING BENEFITS

Everyone can perform magic, everyone can reach his goals, if he is able to think, if he is able to wait, if he is able to fast. -Hermann Hesse, Siddhartha

I have found a multitude of benefits with intermittent fasting. I am feeling the best I've ever felt in my entire life, and it's not just because of losing over 80 pounds. These advantages have helped me stick with intermittent fasting over the course of years, which is a complete departure from any other eating plan I've ever tried. On every other plan, I was counting down the days until I got down to my goal weight, so that I could get back to eating the way I really wanted to eat. But I enjoy intermittent fasting so much, I see no reason to ever stop practicing it. I've found a multitude of benefits, aside from easy, sustainable weight loss.

Improved Mood

Since beginning intermittent fasting, I've found that I don't get hangry, until perhaps right before suppertime. This is completely different than how I felt when I was eating five or six times a day. Back then, I was hangry within a few hours of my last meal. I think my hanger was mostly due to how stressed I became when I had to think about food. And thanks to the advice to eat five or six times a day, I was thinking about food all the time. *What were the right foods to eat, anyway? High protein? High fat? Low carb? Are eggs really bad or good for you? Is a calorie just a calorie? Should I be eating small meals? Or big meals? Or big meals and small snacks?* I had had it rammed in my head that I should be eating every few hours to "rev my metabolism." This also stressed me out, because I felt like each bite was putting more weight on my body, which in hindsight was probably true.

Intermittent fasting made eating much easier. Instead of needing to constantly think about food, there were now large blocks of time where it didn't even need to cross my mind. This put me in a much better mood. And in fact, it was to my benefit if I didn't think about food, because it made the fasting easier. Talk about a win win! I never realized before intermittent fasting, how much my eating, and my being overweight had affected my mood negatively. As I started to lose weight with intermittent fasting, my mood improved even more.

Boundaries With Food

Intermittent fasting has tremendously improved my relationship with food. When I was overweight, I didn't have any boundaries with food. I ate for every reason and no reason: happiness, sadness, boredom, stress, being alone, celebrating with friends. There were no real rules, no true boundaries. Having a boundary with food means basically telling yourself no in some way. The boundary that intermittent fasting sets up is: no eating during this period of time. I do very well with that kind of boundary. Other eating plans set up other types of boundaries that I do not do well with. Setting boundaries around carbs, or calories, or portion sizes drives me crazy. Interestingly, I found that as I set up these time boundaries, I found I had better self-control in general. I learned how to stop eating when I was full. Even better, having boundaries with food also helped me learn how to have boundaries with people.

No Stress Eating

Before intermittent fasting, I had no idea how much of a stress eater I was. I thought that I was eating because I was truly hungry. As it turns out, many times when I was eating, it was simply because I was stressed out. My new reality was that I had a certain window of time in which I could not eat. I had to learn alternative ways to deal with my stress. Things that worked for me were: going for walks, talking it out with my husband, and journaling my thoughts.

Learning About Fake Hunger

Hunger is something you must learn to deal with when you're intermittent fasting. The unexpected lesson I learned was that there are many kinds of hunger. There's boredom hunger, stress hunger, habit hunger, tired hunger, and true hunger. In hindsight I can see that I became overweight mainly due to eating to satisfy all those other fake hungers. Getting that under control has made me a happier person overall, because I'm actually dealing with the causes of my stress, instead of medicating with food.

Learning How To Handle True Hunger

Occasionally I have to deal with true hunger. Sometimes I miscalculate how much I need to eat during my meal. Other times my normal meal time gets pushed later than expected. I have learned how to handle true hunger, and I feel like it has made me stronger as a person. I'm not a slave to my hunger. I can control myself, and this leads to a greater sense of control of my life in general.

Tons Of Energy

I, along with many fellow intermittent fasters I've spoken with, have loads of energy when I'm practicing intermittent fasting. In the beginning, I expected that if I was fasting, I would feel draggy. After all, isn't food supposed to give you energy? But for me, I feel much more energetic during my fasting window. In general I'm an early riser and I feel great all day long. I am sure that having 80 fewer pounds to lug around has improved my energy levels as well.

Increased Focus And Productivity

Since I only need to think about eating once per day, I find that I'm able to focus on everything else and get a whole lot accomplished. Instead of sitting around and thinking about food or eating, I use that time to be productive. Before I started intermittent fasting, I never realized how much time I spent thinking about food, preparing food, eating food, and cleaning up the mess I made from eating food. Now I not only have more time to work, I have more free time to pursue hobbies and interests. As a mom of three, I used to feel like I had no time for myself. When I started fasting, I also started giving myself permission to have "me time" whenever my normal meal times would have been. I used that time to learn new things, and to pursue my interests like reading and drawing.

A Clear Headspace

You know how Steve Jobs always wore black turtlenecks and jeans to save himself from decision fatigue? I've found that intermittent fasting, especially OMAD, provides a similar benefit. Eating requires a lot of decisions. *Should I have scrambled eggs or fried? Should I use butter or oil to fry them in? Should I have two eggs or three? Should I put butter on my toast or jelly? Or both? If I use jelly, should I eat one less egg? Or should I eat one more egg so that my macros are better? Or should I skip the toast altogether?* Fasting saves me a multitude of decisions and gives me a clear headspace.

When I was overweight, I was also constantly thinking about

being overweight. I obsessed about what other people must be thinking about me and how overweight I'd become. My mind was constantly debating what the best way to lose weight and keep it off was, or if I should simply give up on weight loss for good and be happy being overweight. Intermittent fasting solved my weight problem, and it no longer occupies my thoughts.

Cheap

Fasting is cheap. Carbs are cheap. Overall, I am not spending as much money on my own food as I used to, because I simply require less. Also, since I'm not trying to eat a special diet, I don't have to buy special, expensive foods. It also doesn't require any special supplements.

Feels Easy

No other weight loss eating plan I've ever tried has ever felt easy. If it had, I'd probably still be doing that plan. On every other plan, I was always looking forward to the day when I could go back to eating how I wanted, which is of course why I always gained the weight back. But intermittent fasting feels very easy to me. This won't be the case for everyone. My husband, for example, does not find intermittent fasting easy. It suits my personality and strengths.

No Forbidden Foods

It bears repeating that I have no forbidden foods. I eat whatever I want. This has been incredibly freeing. The idea that certain foods should be off limits to me as an overweight person made me feel bitter and deprived. This always led to me overindulging in these forbidden foods. When I finally got rid of the notion of forbidden foods, they truly lost their luster. Counterintuitively, I've found that by allowing myself to have these foods with no limits, I simply eat to satiation and not misery. I also have fewer cravings for what many people would term junk food.

Better Sleep

I sleep much sounder nowadays. I'm sure this is due in part because I've lost a significant amount of weight, but I started noticing this benefit shortly after I started intermittent fasting consistently. In the past I would wake up constantly to go pee. Now I sleep soundly through most nights. I also personally require less sleep now. Sometimes I will wake up after 6 hours of sleep, alert and ready to take on the day. My personal rule is that if I wake up ridiculously early, say 3 or 4 am, I will go ahead and start my day. I'll take a nap if I find I need one. More often than not, I find I do not get drowsy. Not everyone experiences this, but some do.

Food Is Now In Its Rightful Place

When I was overweight, I was kind of obsessed with food. I let it rule my day. I thought about it constantly. I let it ruin my attitude if my mealtime got pushed later than I wanted. Eating was the best, most exciting part of my day. Intermittent fasting revealed how much of a void I was filling with food. Every time I felt stressed, tired, or bored, I ate. I didn't realize I was doing it when I was overweight. Intermittent fasting forced me to adopt more appropriate ways of dealing with each of those feelings. When I was stressed, I started walking, journaling, or talking it out. When I was tired, I took naps or just let myself rest. When I was bored, I started actively pursuing old and new interests.

I Enjoy Food More

Foods taste better to me now. I actually appreciate the tastes of foods that I used to think were bland, like beans. I enjoy the act of eating a meal, because by my one meal, I am actually hungry. I also don't feel all the guilt, stress, and shame I used to feel when I was eating. And thanks to my cheat days, I've learned that I can function around food normally, even when I'm not intermittent fasting. I'm now at peace with food.

Chapter Notes

- I've found intermittent fasting offers many benefits other than weight loss
- Not everyone does great with intermittent fasting
- I have an improved relationship with food
- It feels very easy to me overall
- I've learned how to spot fake hunger
- I sleep better
- I think more clearly thanks to intermittent fasting
- I feel energetic and get a lot more done while I'm fasting

CHAPTER 4: INTERMITTENT FASTING: CHALLENGES

The pessimist sees difficulty in every opportunity. The optimist sees the opportunity in every difficulty. -Winston Churchill

Nothing is without its challenges, and intermittent fasting is no different. While intermittent fasting is the easiest, most sustainable weight loss method I've ever found, I still had to learn to deal with bumps in the road. Fortunately, none of these obstacles was so big that I could not overcome it. Learning how to deal with these challenges has made me a more disciplined person, and I'm better off for it.

Hunger

Hunger is the biggest challenge I faced. I felt so much fear around it. I was afraid if I didn't eat the instant I felt hunger, I would slow down my metabolism and I'd really never be able to lose the weight. I didn't understand this when I was overweight, but the real problem was I was lumping all hunger together. Intermittent fasting taught me there were many kinds of hunger. Nowadays when I feel hunger, I ask myself, are you stressed? Tired? Bored? Is it time for your period? Did you go off plan yesterday? This usually gets to the actual reason I'm feeling hungry.

Stress Hunger

As it turns out, stress hunger was the most common type of hunger I was feeling. Before intermittent fasting, I had no idea how many times I was eating only because I was stressed. I always thought I was truly hungry. But when I started to feel stressed and I was in a fasting window, I couldn't turn to food. Simply not having the option to eat made me start to dig into whether I was actually hungry or not. What I realized was that many times, I was worried about something. I had to learn how to deal with it in a different way. My go to solution is to take a nice long walk. I find that it helps me to think about things more clearly, and puts me in a more positive state of mind. Over time I learned how to talk it out with my husband. Journaling is another tool I keep in my toolbelt. The main thing I've learned is to take action on the thing that's stressing me out, instead of ignoring it.

Fatigue Hunger

Sometimes when I feel hungry, it's not because I'm stressed, but rather because I'm tired. I find this is especially true of nighttime hunger. If I get hungry at night, I just go to bed. Usually I'll fall right to sleep, which means I wasn't hungry. I'm the type of person who has a very hard time falling asleep if I'm truly hungry. If it's in the middle of the day and I'm tired, I take a nap, or just let myself rest. I have learned not to feel guilty for letting myself rest when I need it, because I end up being much more effective if I am firing on all cylinders.

Boredom Hunger

In the beginning, this was a type of hunger I felt a lot. Even though it felt like I was hungry, I was actually just bored. My technique here was to tell myself that if I was still hungry after waiting 30 minutes, I'd allow myself to break my fast early. But to make that 30 minutes pass quickly, I'd go do something else. And when I got busy doing something else, I'd look up two hours later and realize I was no longer hungry. I started to focus on being productive, staying busy, and pursuing my interests actively, rather than sitting around being bored. I also focused on getting my steps in, which also cured my boredom.

Period Hunger

Period hunger is a thing. I've talked to a lot of other women, and many of us get hungry around that time of the month. How I deal with period hunger has evolved over time. In the early days of intermittent fasting, I simply allowed myself to open my eating window earlier. I listened to my body. Eventually I didn't feel the need to open my eating window early, but there was usually one day out of the month that my mood would shift in a bad way. My husband would then bring me a candy bar, and insist that I eat it. We call it my emergency chocolate. I can't remember the last time I required emergency chocolate, but I do still experience a serious mood shift about one day out of every month. I've learned to recognize it for what it is, and this has made it much more bearable. I've also found that it fades within a few hours. To be clear, if I ever really want my emergency chocolate, I will eat it, guilt free. It's just that I haven't needed it for a while.

Habit Hunger

My body quickly adapts to whatever eating schedule I give it. This means that on Monday, the day after my cheat day, I feel hunger at whatever time I ate first on Sunday. Learning to recognize habit hunger for what it is makes it fairly easy to deal with. I generally don't need to do anything for habit hunger. I simply don't eat. I've found the feeling of hunger goes away within 30 minutes to an hour.

True Hunger

I do not experience true hunger during my fasting window on a regular basis. However, in the early days I experienced it more often. It was almost always because I was trying to limit how much food I was eating during my eating window. It went back to getting in a hurry, hoping to speed up my results. Instead, it would backfire, because I would feel hungry during the fasting window, which made it harder to be consistent. In 2016 I was much better (though not perfect!) about being sure to eat to satiation during my eating window. Also, when I went to eating OMAD, I had to learn the line between eating until satiation and overeating. I have found that place now, but it took some experimentation. My process here was to check in with myself after my meal. If I felt overly full, I would not beat myself up for eating too much. I made a mental note that I felt uncomfortably full, and to try at my next meal to pay more attention to how I was feeling. If I ever feel true hunger during my fasting window, I take that as a cue to be sure to eat more during my meal.

Trouble Sleeping

Trouble sleeping was only a problem when I tried to get faster results by eating less during my eating window. I always take restless nights as a signal for the need to eat more. It is very important to eat enough, because when you're tired from not sleeping well, the next day the fasting feels more difficult. When I'm eating the right amount, I sleep very soundly and wake up fully rested.

Nausea, Headaches, Low Energy

If I ever experience nausea, headaches, or low energy, I take it as a signal that I need to eat more during my eating window, and I do. There were times when I got in a hurry with my weight loss in 2016. I'd get impatient, and think that if I'd just eat a little less at my meal, then I would lose weight faster. This always backfired. Since I was not eating to satiation, I would feel hungry all day the next day. On top of that, I also began experiencing the aforementioned unpleasant symptoms. This made fasting feel difficult. I realized quickly that in order for intermittent fasting to work over the long term, I had to eat plenty of food. This felt completely counterintuitive at first, but over time I have found that shortcuts like eating too little delay progress because they cause the plan to feel difficult, which then causes inconsistency.

Nowadays, I have a good handle on how much I need to eat at my meal in order to feel completely satiated, but not overly full. I have found that when I eat to this point, I won't have any negative symptoms in my fasting window, with a few small exceptions. One day out of the month, generally my ovulation time, I will feel a bit of nausea. It's generally only for a few minutes during one day, but it's something I've noticed. Occasionally during my period I notice some nausea before my meal, but this is sporadic, usually once every other month.

Changing Bowel Habits

One difference I noticed when I started OMAD was that my bowel movements were less frequent. When I was overweight and eating 5-6 times a day, I generally had two or more bowel movements a day. With OMAD, I generally find that I go once a day, but there are occasions where I go a day or more between movements. Some other intermittent fasters I've spoken with say they experience more constipation. I do not get constipated, but this could be because I drink coffee three times a day and eat beans rather regularly.

Social Pressure

This is mentally the hardest part of intermittent fasting, in my experience. People who are not familiar with fasting tend to feel very uncomfortable eating in front of someone who is not eating. This can cause an awkward situation, where the person who's eating is urging the person who's fasting to eat. The person who's fasting can feel like she's being sabotaged. I've never been able to convince anyone who's unfamiliar with fasting that I do not mind sitting at the table not eating while they eat. People assume this must be agony for the person who is fasting, and thus they feel very guilty about eating. So, they urge the person to eat, to assuage their own guilt. When you learn to fast, you'll find that it really is no big deal to sit there while people eat, as far as the food and hunger is concerned. Dealing with people is a different matter.

I think it helps to realize that eating is not just about intaking calories. Taking part in a meal with other people is part calorie intake, and part fellowship and celebration. This makes saying no to sharing a meal a bit more complex, because it's not just about the food! Since these times don't come up very often in my life, my rule is to simply eat. Other people find that having a coffee will satisfy the people who are eating. Still others simply say, "I'm not hungry," and they've found that works to stop the urging. There are even some people out there who are able to simply refuse the urge-ers and tell them politely, yet firmly, that they will not be eating at that time. Each person has to figure out which tactic works for them and their personality.

Handling Criticism

With weight loss, you're going to face criticism. You'll get criticized for being too heavy, and you'll get criticized for losing too much. If you're a vegan you'll get criticized for not eating any meat, and if you're a carnivore you'll get criticized for not eating your veggies. The point? You can't please all of the people all of the time. Intermittent fasting is no different. Although fasting is an ancient practice, most people nowadays are not familiar with it. And while eating five or six times a day is the norm now, it wasn't long ago in our history that eating three times or less was the standard. When you divert from the norm, you are bound to come up against criticism.

You have several options here. An informal poll of my YouTube audience shows that the preferred method is to simply not tell people you're fasting. In the beginning, this was my strategy. Even though I was having some success, I knew that early criticism would make me lose confidence in my plan and throw me off track. As my confidence in my plan grew, I began to tell others when they asked me how I was doing it. After I lost 65 pounds and kept it off, I felt confident enough to start my YouTube channel, Six Miles to Supper. At this point, if someone is very critical of my fasting, it doesn't phase me. I know how good I feel, the amazing changes I've made, and how many improvements I've made to my eating in general. To quote Teddy Roosevelt, it's not the critic who counts.

Another option is to try to educate the person who's trying to debate with you. I have found this to be a fairly fruitless endeavor. It's true: those convinced against their will are of the same opinion still. I've found when it comes to weight loss techniques, people generally adopt their chosen diet dogma and hold it with almost the same fervency as their religion. I don't argue religion with people, and I refuse to argue diet dogma as well. However, educating **yourself** about whatever weight loss technique you choose is very important. Even if you can't convince others that it's the best technique for you, it will strengthen your resolve to continue on in the face of criticism.

Lastly, you can choose not to engage with someone who is simply attacking you. There is no requirement that says you must sit and defend your position about your chosen way to eat. You can simply say that you won't discuss it with them, or even walk away if necessary. Having boundaries with people is necessary, and something I'm continually working on. For an excellent guide on this topic, check out the book *Boundaries: When to Say Yes, How to Say No to Take Control of Your Life* by Dr. Henry Cloud and Dr. John Townsend.

Adjusting To The Lifestyle

I pushed my fasting window out so gradually, it never felt like much of an adjustment. I know not everyone has the patience to go so gradually, so I ask every intermittent faster I can about their adjustment time frame. The most common physical adjustment is simply learning to deal with hunger. Most people report that even when they've aggressively pushed out their window, going from eating 5 or 6 times a day straight to OMAD, the adjustment period is no longer than 3 weeks. Most report even shorter adjustment periods.

The greater adjustment, in my opinion, is the mental one. To do this on a daily basis, consistently, requires a mental shift. This is about lifestyle change. It also requires learning how to deal with all the various kinds of hunger in ways other than by eating. It's about learning to restructure your days so that they don't revolve around food. It means that you'll have to adjust to not having a meal or two a day with your family. You have to learn how to be okay with being different in this area of your life. I have found a major benefit of my weekly cheat day is that it gives me one day of complete normalcy with my family.

Plateaus

Weight loss plateaus happen on every single weight loss plan, and intermittent fasting is no different. It can be very frustrating to only eat once a day, and still have the scale stall out for weeks at a time. Yes, that's happened to me, especially as my BMI got into the normal range. I have found that if you give the scale two months, it eventually catches back up with your efforts. It just takes a big dose of stubborness and consistency over time. Whenever I'm going through a plateau, I check in with myself. I ask myself if I'm sticking to my plan. If the answer is no, I work on being more consistent. If the answer is yes, I ask myself if I'm stressed. If the answer is yes, I try to actively eliminate that stress, which usually means taking some sort of action. For example, if the stress is about money, I work on bringing in some extra income. Usually inconsistency or stress is the cause of my plateau. But other times, there doesn't seem to be a reason. So, I wait it out. I don't change my plan. I don't try longer fasts to get the scale moving. I don't take cheat day away. I don't change my plan, because I really like my plan. It feels really easy. I know myself well enough to know that if I start tinkering with it, I'll end up making it harder and harder, and eventually I'll give up. I've resisted the urge to ever change my plan since January 2016, and I've been able to lose over 80 pounds and keep it off.

Chapter Notes

- Every plan has challenges, and intermittent fasting is no different
- Learning how to deal with hunger is the biggest physical challenge
- Dealing with the social pressure to eat is the greatest mental challenge
- In general, negative symptoms are a signal that you should eat more
- Intermittent fasting is a deviation from the norm. Expect criticism.
- Plateaus happen. Stay stubborn and consistent. They will break.

CHAPTER 5: GETTING STARTED WITH INTERMITTENT FASTING

The scariest moment is always just before you start. -Stephen King

When you're first starting out with intermittent fasting, you'll probably wonder exactly how you should implement it. It can be overwhelming, and even scary. You'll have a million questions. How long of a fast should you start out with? When should your fasting window be? What is the optimal time to fast? To eat? How aggressively should you push out your fasting window? Ultimately, the way to get over these fears is to simply take action. There are no real right answers, there is no one best way. Instead of trying to find the perfect plan, it's better to just get started and then iterate from there. You can make it as hard or as easy on yourself as you like in the beginning. The key is to be willing to experiment with your plan and not give up. When I made my plan, I took the very easy route, which I will describe below. Although my results were slower, I believe this path had some distinct advantages.

The Path Of Least Resistance

In December 2014 I started out with a fasting window of about 8 hours. Yes, that means I slept through it. I'd tell myself that I couldn't eat after 10pm, and I had to wait to eat breakfast until after 6am. I was learning how to put time boundaries around food. I slowly pushed breakfast later and later, until eventually lunch was my first meal. Then I started pushing lunch later and later. In 2015, I was hesitant to do fasts of longer than 14 hours consistently. Eventually I decided it was a bigger risk to remain overweight, so I started to experiment with longer fasts. I eventually read that women could safely practice fasts of longer than 14 hours, which confirmed my own experience. I found I felt fantastic: not only was my weight coming down, but my energy levels were way up.

By the beginning of 2016, I was at about a 16:8 fast. Generally I'd stop eating at 10pm, and not eat until 2pm. I had no rules about how many meals or snacks to have during my eating window. What it generally looked like was: I was good and hungry when my window opened, so I'd eat a good sized late lunch. Then I wouldn't feel hungry until supper. Most of the time I'd eat a snack right as my eating window was closing, to ensure that my fasting window felt as easy as possible the next day. I gradually pushed my window out, usually only by 30 minute increments. By March 2016, I was at a 20:4 fast. I kept pushing my window out further because I thought it would make me lose weight faster.

Then, the stomach virus hit our household. I was so nervous about eating one day that I really just couldn't force myself to eat until suppertime. That happened for several days in a row (I never got sick, thankfully, I just used to be super-afraid of the stomach virus). I realized that I didn't die when I only ate once a day. In fact, I felt really good when I only ate once. I had tons of energy, and even more free time! I also dropped 6 pounds that week. I immediately started googling "is it okay to only eat once a day?" That's when I ran across an article about OMAD. I figured as long as I was feeling good, and the scale kept moving in the right direction, I would try it.

I think it is important to note something here. If you compare my rate of weight loss over time, you'll find that it averaged one pound a week, whether I was doing a shorter fast, longer fasts, or even OMAD. The thing I liked about OMAD was the simplifying of my life. I think it's a mistake to aggressively push out your fasting window in the hopes you will have faster results. Instead, focus on being consistent with fasting during your fasting window, and eating during your eating window. If you find you are not losing weight at all, despite being consistent with your window, then slowly push out your window until you get the results you're looking for.

Slow Vs Fast

One huge advantage, I believe, is that as I incorporated fasting into my life slowly, it became a way of life for me. Fasting is a deviation from the norm in our society. It helped it to feel more normal to me since I took it so slowly. It deeply ingrained the habit of fasting within me. Fasting is a skill, and the more you practice it, the better you get. This made me a lot more consistent than I would have been, had I tried to go faster. This is probably due to my own personal temperament, but I think it is worth mentioning.

This also meant that fasting always felt relatively easy to me (especially when I learned how to deal with various types of hunger).I have seen others aggressively push out their window, but find that they're struggling with consistency. If you find that happening to you, I urge you to make your plan easier. I believe this has been crucial to my long term success with both losing the weight and keeping it off. When something feels easy, you can keep at it forever. If something feels hard, you can keep it up for a while, but usually you get tired of it being so hard, and you quit. Or at least, that's what I do.

Can you go faster? Sure! I've talked to some people who go straight from eating five or six times a day to OMAD with no issues at all. And if that feels easy to you, and you find you can be super consistent with it, and you're feeling awesome, I say more power to you! But, if you find you're not able to be consistent, and it's feeling hard, my advice would be to give yourself permission to take the slow and easy route. It works too. I'm proof of that. And, you might even find that it is faster than the harder way, because you can be more consistent right off the bat. But before you begin intermittent fasting, you need to figure out your goal and a plan.

Set Your Goals

It's important to begin with the end in mind. Figure out where you want to go with your weight loss. When you pick a number, have a reason for it. If you don't know why you want to be down to a certain weight, you're going to struggle to stay motivated. If you have no idea what a healthy weight for you is, I have found that the Body Mass Index is a nice guideline, and it's also helpful because it gives you a rather broad range. You might not know exactly where you want to be, but it helps to know the general range you'd like to be in. Staying flexible with your goals is important too. You may find, as you reach your goal weight, that you want to lose more. Conversely, you might find that you are happy at a weight higher than your original goal weight. The important thing to focus on is how you're feeling about your weight, and where you feel happiest. Remember also that you have the option of maintaining for a while, and then losing more weight if you so desire. You're in control of your journey.

For example, at 5'6" a normal weight for me is between 115 and 154. My original goal was to get down to 154, but I found that when I got to 157 I was very happy with how I felt and how I looked. Also, at that point, the holidays were upon me, and I wasn't sure how that would go. I decided to maintain for a while. After maintaining that easily for almost a year, I decided I wanted to be firmly in that normal BMI range, and since then I've lost 17 more pounds.

Form Your Plan

I've found it's important to have a written plan of some sort. If you're on a written plan, it is then possible to ask yourself if you are sticking to your plan. In so doing, you can hold yourself accountable. It's impossible to hold yourself accountable if you don't have a plan. A written plan also makes it possible to track your data and test the plan to see if it is working or not. It's too easy to let feelings lead you off course. Sometimes it *feels* like the plan is not working, when the numbers tell an entirely different story.

But perhaps you hate the idea of being on a written plan. Maybe you're afraid that it will feel really constrictive. The good news here is that you can make the plan have exactly the rules you want it to have. You can write a lot of freedom into your plan. You want to eat a whole bag of peanut butter M&Ms every Tuesday at 2pm? It's your plan! Let your imagination run wild. Remember, this is just an experiment. Consider the following when writing out your plan:
- What types of foods you're allowing yourself to have
- What kind of exercise you're committing to, if any
- How many days of the week you will be intermittent fasting
- Whether or not you'll take a cheat day

Consider Your Personality

While you're forming your plan, It's important to think about your personality. One major thing that I didn't consider in the beginning of my weight loss journey was my introversion. As an introvert, I get energy from being alone. Being in a large group of people is exhausting and quite often stressful. As it turns out, a lot of weight loss advice is geared towards extroverted people, and doesn't really gel with introverts. For example, the common advice is, start going to the gym every day. But going to a loud gym with lots of people can be taxing on an introvert. We can then beat ourselves up for not consistently going, when in fact, we would be much more consistent if we found something that was a better fit.

I found that walking inside my house was a perfect match for my personality. I also realized that I tended to overeat at social events, because I felt uncomfortable. I started turning down invitations to certain events that I knew I would not enjoy. For events I choose to attend, I intentionally decide to eat at the event, because I know that when people are urging me to eat, I prefer to go ahead and eat. I also make it a point during the event to check in with myself about how I'm feeling. I am aware that I'll have a tendency to eat simply because I'm feeling uncomfortable. When I find that is happening, I give myself a break by finding a nice quiet corner, or even going to the restroom and hanging out there for a few minutes. While you are forming your plan, start considering those times in your life when it will make sense for you to go off plan.

What Would It Look Like If It Were Easy?

Ask yourself what weight loss would look like if it were easy. You don't get a badge for making this plan hard. Consider putting in a weekly cheat day. As an example, my plan looked like this:
- Intermittent fasting 6 days a week, eating whatever and however much I want
- Walk 6 miles a day
- Cheat day on Sunday

I know. It's counterintuitive to focus on making something easy, especially if you are a high achiever. We tend to think hard equals big results, easy equals lack of effort. But think in terms of working smarter, not harder. If you make a plan that's really hard, and that you can't stick with over the long term, you're planning for eventual failure. Instead, think of the things you can stick with forever, if necessary. That's the key to long term sustainability.

Track It

Decide how you will track your results. I have found weighing daily and keeping track of my 7 day average to be the best way for me. The scale, while certainly not perfect, is an easy tool to use and a hard thing to cheat. The scale can provide you with daily data, and over time gives an accurate answer as to whether your weight loss plan is working or not.

Test Your Plan

Now comes the fun part. Commit to your plan and simply stick to it for the next six weeks. Track using whatever method you chose. Be sure to put a reminder on your calendar for when the six weeks is up. Then sit down with your data and look at the results. It's important to not only look at pounds lost. Also consider things like:
- Energy levels
- Overall mood
- Perceived level of effort
- Consistency

If your results were good, it's feeling easy, you're feeling great, and you're being consistent, I say your plan is a winner. If you're having trouble with consistency, try making your plan easier, and give it another go. It's all about tweaking your plan, experimenting, and finding what works for you.

How To Begin Fasting

Getting started with intermittent fasting is easy. It's important to consider your strengths, your schedule, and daily life when you start the process of intermittent fasting in order to set yourself up for success.

Step 1: Pick Your Fasting Window Length

Don't overthink this. You're just learning how to put a time boundary around food here. If you're a grazer by nature, like me, you might want to start out with something short, like 8 hours. If 8 hours feels too long, shorten it to whatever feels doable to you. In the beginning you're just learning the skill of fasting. You probably won't have any noticeable weight loss with intermittent fasting until you reach a 12 hour fast. Most people report the best, most consistent results when the fasting window is 16 hours or more. That being said, everyone is different, so you just need to find what works for you.

Step 2: Pick Your Fasting Window Time

Again, look at your daily life. When is it the easiest for you to not eat? For me, breakfast was the meal that I could skip the easiest. Most of the time I didn't actually feel hungry. I just felt obligated to eat because that's what all the weight loss experts told me I should be doing. Once you've picked your fasting window time, simply put it into practice. Each day (except for cheat day, which I highly recommend), don't eat during your fasting window time.

Step 3: Work On Consistency

This is perhaps the most important, but overlooked step. People get so focused on making the fasting window longer and longer that they're not paying attention to how consistent they can be with it. Try the fasting window length and time you picked for a week and see how it feels. Are you able to not eat during your fasting window? How easy does it feel? If it feels easy and you're having results, don't change anything. There is no need to make it harder on yourself. If you're able to stay consistent, but it doesn't truly feel easy, stay on this step for a while longer. Most likely, within a week or so, your body will adjust to this window, and it will feel easy. If it's feeling easy, you're being super consistent, and you're still not seeing results, then move on to the next step.

Step 4: Lengthen Your Window, If Necessary

When you lengthen your window, you can do it gradually. An additional half hour or an hour is plenty. After you've lengthened it, practice staying consistent with it. If at any point you find you're inconsistent, make your fasting window a little shorter. Work on consistency, and then lengthen by a bit. Most people find that when they are consistent with intermittent fasting, they lose weight. The snag most people hit is that they fail to be consistent. I have found that consistency is tied to difficulty. Easy plan equals lots of consistency, hard plan equals lots of off plan days.

Stick To Your Plan

Once you have tested your plan, it feels easy, and you're having results, it's simply time to commit to it for the long haul. You might find you have to tweak it, especially if it starts to feel too hard. I never had to tweak the plan I formed in January 2016, but I did have to start forming a code for myself about when to go off plan. This was formed over time, as random situations came up. Your life and your code will probably look much different than mine, but the important thing to do is to realize right now that life happens. Vacations happen. **You will need to go off plan on occasion.** Start thinking now about how you'll handle those things, and you'll save yourself a lot of stress later on. (More on this in the chapter about going off plan.)

When To Stop Losing

How do you decide when to stop losing? That's a fantastic question, and it's one only you can answer. I believe each person has their own weight that they feel the best at. Some people don't mind being a bit heavier. Some want an excellent physique.

And some just want to be at a normal BMI. It all comes down to what would make you happiest. I urge you not to worry about what other people think. Instead, focus on your own feelings about yourself. Learning how to be happy with my body, and all its imperfections, has been a slow and steady process. I remind myself that in college when I was at a healthy weight, I was obsessively critical of what I looked like in photographs. I was always focused on my stomach not being flat, or my face not looking thin. Nowadays, I focus on the positive. If I catch myself focusing on the negative, I remind myself that it's a road to chronic unhappiness.

Personally, I'm completely happy in the 140 range, and I don't care if I lose more. But I also love my plan. And currently I'm still losing, though very slowly at this point (a third of a pound a week on average.) I have a feeling that my weight loss will level off at some point and my current plan will simply keep me maintaining at a healthy weight. If I continue to lose until I get on the low end of the normal range, I will open up my eating window a bit, as I have no desire to be underweight. According to my research, being underweight is as dangerous as being obese.

Beware The Intermittent Fasting Police

If you hang out online with other intermittent fasters, you're eventually going to deal with the intermittent fasting police. These are well-intentioned people who believe in their heart of hearts that it is their job to enforce the Rules of Intermittent Fasting. If you choose to have cream in your coffee, they'll warn you that it's knocking you out of the fasted state. If you decide to give yourself a shorter fasting window, they'll preach to you that you are missing out on the benefits of longer fasting. I've found it's best to simply thank these individuals for their advice, and then go on my merry way.

Chapter Notes

- Going gradually with intermittent fasting has many benefits
    - It feels easier
    - You'll probably be more consistent
    - It will seem less weird
- Most people don't notice weight loss until 12 hour fasts or longer, some not until 16 or more
- Longer fasting windows don't necessarily lead to faster weight loss
- It's best to find the fasting window that you enjoy most, because that is the one you'll be most consistent with
- When choosing your window, set yourself up for success by putting your fasting window during the times it's easiest for you not to eat
- Only lengthen your window after you're consistent with your current window
- Write out a plan for your weight loss
    - Make rules for yourself that sound easy to follow
    - Write some freedom into your plan
    - Commit to it for 6 weeks and track your results
    - Tweak if necessary
    - Commit for the long term
    - Accept that you will occasionally need to go off plan

CHAPTER 6: GOING OFF PLAN

Fall down seven times. Get up eight. - Japanese proverb

I am not perfect on this plan. *Spoiler alert!* You are not going to be perfect on your plan. Repeat after me: life happens. I will occasionally go off plan. I am not perfect. No one is perfect.

If you're a perfectionist like I was, you'll balk at that statement. But the sooner you can come to terms with the fact that no one is perfect, everyone messes up occasionally, and life just happens, the better off you're going to be. In the past, I would get frustrated by occasions that would come up that would take me off my plan. I would stress over how to handle it. Eventually I heard some really good advice on Jaime Masters' podcast, *The Eventual Millionaire*. She said that if you find yourself coming up against a similar situation over and over again, you should make a rule for yourself on how to handle that situation. Then, from that point forward, you have a predetermined decision, and you don't have to make it over and over again. I looked at this as a way to form a code for myself.

My Code

My code for going off plan has many rules, and it was built over time, based on situations that continually came up in my life. Your life is very different than mine, so your rules will be different. But to give you an idea of what it can look like, here's a partial look at my code:

- If I attend an event (such as a wedding or a party or a family get together), I will eat.
- I will not limit portion sizes or types of food in any event. I always eat ad libitum.
- If my child makes something and it is outside my window (such as a dessert several hours after dinner), I will eat it.
- If my husband asks me to have popcorn with him as a late night snack, I will.
- If my husband asks me to have a glass of wine with him, I will.
- If I am on a "me time" outing, I will eat if I so desire.
- If it is a family fun event, such as getting ice cream in the middle of the day, I will eat.
- If I have a business lunch, I will eat.
- If I go off plan for any reason during the week, I still take my cheat day as normal on Sunday.

I stick to my code stringently. You'll notice that I always take the easier choice, which is to eat. If one of these scenarios pops up, I will still additionally eat my usual meal at supper time. I'm all about making life easy on myself. I should also note that my code is always subject to change. This has yet to happen, but if I find that the code is making me go off plan 10% of the time or more (almost once a week), AND I find that it is negatively affecting my weight, then I will make a small change in the code.

Holidays

The holidays are a special time, and they're centered around eating. I generally take holidays completely off. For me, this includes: Fourth of July, Halloween, Thanksgiving Day, New Year's Eve, and New Year's Day. Christmastime is a different matter altogether.

After Thanksgiving, there tends to be a constant stream of holiday baking, parties, get togethers, and celebrations until the New Year. Again, I tend to think in terms of making it super easy on myself. Brace yourself for the next sentence. I accept that I will gain some weight.

I know. I know. You don't want to gain any weight. But here's the thing. I believe life is about living. And Christmastime is special. It's basically a month centered around food and family and fun. My general plan for December is to:
- Bake special treats and enjoy them with my kids
- Share meals with other families that we might not see for the rest of the year
- Sit and watch our favorite Christmas movies and eat popcorn and cookies
- Continue to weigh every single day
- Continue to track my 7 day average

This is what I did in 2015, 2016, and 2017. The most I gained? 3.2 pounds. That happened in 2017. It took me a month to get back to where I was before the holidays. Was it worth it? You bet!

Vacations

Vacations used to fill me with dread, but not anymore. There is power in being intentional. I still don't have a cut and dried plan for vacations, because it depends on the vacation. But I always go in with a plan. Sometimes the plan is to be completely off plan the entire time. Other times the plan is to push my eating window as late as possible each day. Other times, I simply stay on my regular plan. One thing that might seem odd, but that actually gives me a lot of peace, is to have my scale with me so that I can continue to weigh. I really like knowing where my weight is. I've also gone on vacation without the scale and I've been fine too. Ultimately, I'm at peace because I know that even if I gain some weight during the vacation, I can go right back to eating OMAD and the weight will come right back off.

Intentionality

The most important theme here is intentionality. There is a big difference in the mental consequences, depending on whether you were intentional or not. If you don't intend to go off plan, but you end up going off plan, there's guilt and frustration. But if your plan is to go off plan, it's empowering. You made a decision, and you stuck with it. Even though your decision was to eat, it gives you a sense of control.

Getting Back On Plan

I remember the first time I went off plan for several days on purpose. We were on vacation and I wanted to fully enjoy the time with my family, meaning that I wanted to eat whenever they did. I felt so much fear at first. *What if this is it? What if I go off plan and never get back on plan again? What if this is the turning point, the return to my old ways?* But then I remembered that every Monday was like getting back from vacation. My weekly cheat day on Sunday was basically a vacation day where I ate whatever and whenever. And every Monday, like clockwork, I got back on plan.

If your plan feels easy enough, I believe it will be easy to get back on plan. If you find yourself resistant to getting back on plan, it's a red flag. **Danger, Will Robinson!** It means your plan is too difficult. It's not sustainable. You need to tweak your plan so that it's one that you don't mind being on, one that you, I daresay, enjoy. Do not beat yourself up or panic if you realize you hate your plan. Instead, look at it as an opportunity to improve. Be grateful that you've made the realization, and take the steps to tweak your plan to make it exactly what you want it to look like. It also helps to think about your why. Why are you wanting to lose weight in the first place?

Chapter Notes

- Accept up front that you will need to go off plan from time to time
- After you form your plan and you start practicing it

consistently also start forming a code
  - Your code is for scenarios that come up from time to time
  - Consider making your default behavior the easiest choice to make
  - Remember that you can always tweak the code if you find it is too lax
- Be intentional with holidays. It's okay to take them off
- Be intentional with vacations. Go in with a plan. Enjoy yourself.
- There is power that comes with being intentional, even if your decision is to intentionally go off plan
- Getting back on plan is easy if your plan is easy
  - If you have trouble getting back on plan, make your plan easier
  - Consider implementing a weekly cheat day in order to consistently practice going off plan and getting back on plan

CHAPTER 7: MY DAILY ROUTINE

We are what we repeatedly do. Excellence, then, is not an act, but a habit. -Will Durant

So what does my own daily routine with OMAD look like? Every day is somewhat different. Some days my walk is split up into short bursts throughout the day, sometimes it's one long 6 mile walk. My coffee times vary, based on what my schedule for the day holds. My suppertime is sometimes earlier in the evening, sometimes later. I'm very laid back about the whole thing, really. But, there are some features that remain constant:

Weighing

Every morning, right after I wake up and use the restroom, I weigh myself. I log that number into my Fitbit app so that I have a physical record of it. I only weigh once a day. Weight fluctuates throughout the day, and I've found it's quite pointless and only stressful to weigh more than once. However, once a day is important, as it keeps me accountable to my plan on a daily basis.

Eating

Ever since April of 2016, when I've been in weight loss mode, I've eaten OMAD Monday through Saturday. I do occasionally go off plan, on purpose, which is detailed in Chapter 6. I have chosen supper as my one meal, and that is the only time I eat. I sit down with my family at the supper table, and we all eat together, no television or devices. I eat however much I want. I eat whatever I want. This is generally just normal food that any family eats: spaghetti with jarred sauce, rice and beans, tacos, hamburgers. It's just your typical American family fare. It seems like the list of "bad foods" changes from year to year. I've officially given up on paying attention to it. I try to enjoy all things, from grains and meats, to veggies and fruits, to sweets and dairy and fats. If I am craving a certain thing during the day, I have it at my meal. To reiterate, I like big portions. I usually eat 2 or 3 platefuls of food. I simply eat until I feel good and full, but not overly full. When supper is over, I stand up from the table, and I don't eat again until the next day at supper time.

Coffee

I drink coffee with half and half three times a day, every day of the week. I do not measure the amounts, but it's about 12 oz of coffee and 2-3 tablespoons of half and half each time. The half and half is full fat half and half. Fat free half and half has corn syrup in it, so I do not use it. Generally I have a cup of coffee upon waking, another cup an hour or so later, and then an afternoon cup. If I am craving more, I'll drink it guilt free. But usually, I stick with three because I tend to feel more anxiety if I have more. I drink regular coffee only, never decaf, simply because I don't see the point. I'm the type of person who can drink coffee right before bed and fall sound asleep.

Exercise

I walk six miles every single day of the week, which is 14,000 steps on my Fitbit. I count every step I take that day, incidental steps from life in general, and my longer walks. When I lived in a traditional house, I did all of my steps in my house. Since becoming a full-time RVer, I get my steps in by going on hikes or just walking around outside. However, on bad weather days, I get my steps inside our 31' Class C Winnebago. I get my steps in extremely consistently, with perhaps 2 missed days in a year. I walk slowly, at a pace of about 3 miles per hour, which is therefore about two hours of walking every day.

Cheat Day

Sunday is my cheat day, or my day off from fasting, if you prefer. I eat whatever I want, whenever I want, however many times I want, throughout the day. Some cheat days that means I eat as soon as I wake up, and generally eat like a hobbit for the rest of the day. Other days I eat breakfast and don't get hungry again until dinner. **The point of cheat day is not to overeat.** The point is simply to eat whatever you want whenever you feel like it. One regular feature of my cheat day is that I eat breakfast. My husband started a tradition years ago of making homemade from scratch, chocolate chip pancakes for us on Sunday mornings. Cheat days make enjoying this special treat with my family a guilt free experience. I credit cheat days as a major component to my weight loss success. They are so important, I've devoted the entire next chapter to them.

Chapter Notes

- My daily routine is laid back as far as the daily structure
- I weigh first thing every morning
- My OMAD is supper
    - I eat whatever and however much I want
    - I try to eat to complete satiation, but not so much that I feel overly full
    - I do this Monday through Saturday
- I walk 6 miles per day
- Sunday is my cheat day
    - The only rule is to eat whatever I want and whenever I want
    - The goal is not to overeat, but to simply have freedom

CHAPTER 8: CHEAT DAY

Successful design is not the achievement of perfection but the minimization and accommodation of imperfection. -Henry Petroski

Yes, cheat day is so important, it gets its own chapter. Why? Because this is a part of my plan that has been **critical** to my success. Many people I talk to are afraid to take a cheat day, and my goal with this chapter is to allay those fears, once and for all. I have found cheat days are an awesome tool for weight loss, even though they seem totally counterintuitive. Since January 2016, my cheat day has been each week on Sunday. I never take cheat days away from myself, period. I see a lot of people who refuse to take a cheat day, because they are convinced they'll reach their goals faster if they don't. Sadly, I've also seen a lot of these same people giving up, or failing to be consistent and getting poor results. Far from slowing my progress, I believe cheat days helped me achieve my goals faster.

What Is Cheat Day?

Cheat day is a day with one rule: you eat what you want, when you want, however many times you want, throughout the day. Some people prefer to call it a day off. You eat ad libitum. When I first heard of the concept of cheat day, I thought it sounded too good to be true. I believed cheat days would screw up all the progress I made during the week. Then I read that cheat days actually helped people stick with their weight loss eating plans. I also read that they could help with metabolism, which is something I was super paranoid about with intermittent fasting. As it turns out, the science behind the metabolic benefits of cheat days is shaky at best, but I have found many other benefits.

Benefits

Plan Adherence

In the beginning, when I was learning how to fast, there were times when I would crave certain foods. My daughter would be in the kitchen making cinnamon toast for breakfast. If you're new to this, you have no clue how delicious buttery cinnamon toast smells during a fast. The problem was, of course, I couldn't eat the toast then, because it was during my fasting window. While it's true that I could have some in my eating window, it didn't always work out that way. By the time my window opened it was lunch time and I wanted traditional lunch time food. And, when I started eating OMAD, I found certain foods just didn't make sense at my one meal. A good example is turkey sandwiches. I don't really want those at supper time, but I want them in my life sometimes. If I did not have a cheat day in which I could satisfy these cravings, I would start to feel deprived. The plan would start to feel hard, and eventually I'd go off plan. Instead, I never have to wait longer than a week to satisfy my cravings, which helps me stick to my plan very consistently.

When I was forming my plan in January 2016, I realized there was one thing that was throwing me off with intermittent fasting consistently: our pancake breakfast on Sunday mornings. So every Sunday, I was going off plan. And then I'd sort of try to fast the rest of the day, but I found it difficult since it was our day off from work. When I was working out my plan, I realized that a cheat day made perfect sense for Sunday. I could simply take the day off on purpose. As an added bonus, I realized our extended family gatherings tended to happen on Sundays as well, which meant that I no longer had to deal with the stress of feeling like I was being inconsistent when I inevitably ate at these events.

Relationship With Food

By allowing myself a day off from fasting with no other rules, I've actually improved my relationship with food. I've learned that even on a day with complete freedom, I eat to satiation, not misery. While I eat whatever, whenever, and however much I want, I find that I'm eating normal amounts, and generally eating normal foods. In short, I've learned to trust myself around food.

Cheat days in the beginning had a lot more junk food, but since they were not forbidden, I started to be able to actually figure out if I enjoyed them or if I was eating them to try to prove a point. I found there are certainly some things I still enjoy (Double Stuf Oreos, I'm looking at you), but I end up eating a normal amount and not feeling miserable. I found other foods that I used to find so incredibly tempting, like chocolate chip granola bars, were actually not enjoyable, so I no longer eat them. This has been a process, but it has happened for me over time.

A Cure For My Perfectionism

I'm a recovering perfectionist. I have this tendency to be an all or nothing type person. In the past, if I screwed up just once, I tended to quit forever on the thing. This was true of anything in life, but here's how it looked when it came to weight loss: I'd be on a diet, but the first time I cheated on it, I quit it for good, because I had messed up my streak. Or if it was exercise, say running 3 miles a day, I'd do it every day for months. And then, if I missed one day, I just gave up, and would not get back to it. Cheat days prevent me from ever thinking I can be perfect with intermittent fasting. It breaks my streak every week, and I find it enormously helpful. In school I was a straight A student, and anything lower sent me spiraling. But with this plan, I can only be a B+ intermittent fasting student at best. I have found this incredibly freeing, and it keeps me very consistent.

Learning how to get back on plan

Everyone goes off plan at some point. Life happens. Sit and think for a moment. Have you ever stayed on any plan 100% of the time? Think about vacations. Birthdays. Holidays. Sicknesses. Celebrations. Times of stress or grieving. In general, these are the times when people go off plan. Learning how to get back on plan is a skill. The problem with these life events is that they're random and usually spaced far apart, so you can't practice getting off plan and getting back on based solely on these times. For me, cheat days have been a weekly practice of going off plan, and learning how to get back on plan. Because of this, I have no trouble getting back on plan when I come back from vacations or other times of being off plan.

A Day of Normalcy
I've practiced intermittent fasting for years now, and even though it's normal for me, it's not normal when compared to how my husband and kids eat. It's nice to have one day out of the week that I eat all of my meals with them. And they enjoy this too. The evolution of my own cheat day has shown me that even when I have no rules at all, I can eat like a regular person and not binge. And while I don't think that I'll ever go back to eating three meals a day as a way of life, it helps me to know that I could trust myself to do so.

Makes intermittent fasting easier
Cheat days make intermittent fasting easier, in the beginning especially. When intermittent fasting is new, it may feel hard, if not physically, mentally. A time restriction is still a restriction. It's a mental challenge to restrict yourself. Knowing that come cheat day, you can eat whatever you want, whenever you want, can get you through those occasional challenging days.

Downsides

Temporary weight gain
Yes, when you have a cheat day, especially if you eat lots of salty

and sugary foods, water weight gain will happen. That's what happens to me. And the weight can be significant. Two weeks ago, my weight fluctuated up five pounds overnight, because of some cheat day food that had lots of soy sauce. And you know what happened? Two days later my weight was right back down where it had been. What happens to many people is that they finally try a cheat day, have water weight gain, and swear off cheat days forever. And sadly, they miss the amazing benefits of cheat day. In one way, I almost look at this temporary weight gain as a benefit. I used to think every upward fluctuation meant I was on the wrong path. Now I have learned that fluctuations really don't matter and they can be very arbitrary. It's more important to pay attention to the trend of your weight over time, rather than the daily fluctuations.

Hunger The Day After
Most people experience more hunger than usual the day after cheat day. I think of it as habit hunger, not true hunger. My body quickly remembers the time it expects to be fed. If I feed it at 9am on Sunday, it thinks it should be fed at 9am on Monday. Luckily, this also means that when I don't feed it until 6:30pm on Monday, it doesn't expect food until 6:30pm on Tuesday. Learning to deal with hunger is a skill, and after you've done intermittent fasting for a while, this really isn't an issue. In the beginning, I suggest keeping very busy the day after cheat day. Just expect the hunger to show up, and mentally prepare yourself to deal with it.

Cheat Day The Wrong Way

There is one wrong way to do cheat day. That's when you do it half way. I did this at certain points in my journey. I'd decide to "be good" on cheat day. I wouldn't eat that piece of chocolate. I wouldn't fix myself that sandwich or have that random helping of potato chips that I really wanted to have. And then you know what would happen? During the week, I found myself being tempted to cheat during the fasting window. *Hey, I was good on cheat day, so I can have a few bites of this sandwich now during my fasting window.* When I started seeing this line of thinking show up, I immediately made the decision to always do cheat day right. I never deny myself anything on cheat day. I found it made me extremely consistent through the week.

Cheat Day In Real Life

Cheat day is a complete break from fasting for me. I generally wake up early without an alarm, and enjoy my morning routine with coffee, reading, and journaling. When the rest of my family wakes up, my husband starts making the pancake breakfast. I usually enjoy 3 or 4 delicious chocolate chip from scratch pancakes with real butter and maple syrup with another cup of coffee. By lunchtime, I'm ready to eat again, and I'll usually have some leftovers from the previous week. In the afternoon I'll usually have a snack. I make it a point to eat at suppertime. When I first started doing cheat day, I would be full around 4:00 or 4:30, and I wouldn't eat again for the rest of the day. This meant a longer fast than usual on Monday, a day where I already felt more hunger than normal because of habit hunger. After I realized what I was doing, I decided to always make it a point to eat at supper, or even right before bed, so that fasting is easier the next day.

Chapter Notes

- It's normal to feel afraid of cheat day at first
- Cheat day will not undo all of your progress throughout the week
    - You will gain water weight, but the weight will leave within a couple of days
- Cheat day benefits:
    - Better plan adherence
    - Improved relationship with food
    - Deters perfectionism
    - Teaches you how to get back on plan

- It's a day of normalcy
        - Makes intermittent fasting easier, especially in the beginning
        - It helps you to trust yourself around food
- Cheat day downsides:
    - Temporary weight gain
    - More hunger during the fasting window the next day
- Do not try to "be good" on cheat day. Give yourself exactly what you want.
- Cheat days are simply a break from fasting days for me
    - I eat whatever I want
    - I eat whenever I want
    - I eat as many times as I want
    - I don't end up bingeing on foods
    - I always eat something at suppertime or right before bed so that fasting on Monday is as easy as possible

CHAPTER 9: INTERMITTENT FASTING AND EXERCISE

"It is easier to act yourself into a new way of thinking, than it is to think yourself into a new way of acting." -Millard Fuller

When I was forming my plan in January 2016, I figured I should make exercise a part of it. I'm the type of person who often forgets what day it is, and so I figured it would be much easier on myself if I chose something I could do every single day. I didn't want to worry about leg day or rest days or keep up with how many reps at what weight. So I chose to walk six miles every day.

Why Move?

This is a fair question. One of my favorite sayings is that you can't outrun your fork. I believe it's true. Overall, if you want to lose weight, you have to change the eating in some way. I've talked to many people who are frustrated because they've started walking consistently, but haven't lost any weight. It appears to me that if you're going to change one side of the equation, change the eating side. I'll be the first one to point out that many people have had lots of success with intermittent fasting while doing no exercise at all. None. Some people point out that exercise can increase your appetite, so the increase in calorie burn (approximately 450 calories based on my pace and weight) might just get cancelled out by the fact that I'll eat more during my eating window. I know this. And yet I keep walking those six miles every day. Why would I do such a thing? I have many good reasons.

Easier Fasting

In the beginning of my intermittent fasting journey, I was a stress eater. And a boredom eater. I was a grazer. I was a I-don't-want-the-few-bites-left-on-my-kid's-lunch-plates-to-go-to-waste eater. But since I was intermittent fasting, there was a chunk of time in which I could not be this type of eater. And I needed something else to do with my time. Having the goal of six miles gave me something to do during the fasting window. Over time, I learned that I could also fill my fasting window with all sorts of hobbies, chores, and work in general, but in the beginning, getting more steps in was my go-to.

Mood

It's almost impossible to be in a bad mood after you've walked six miles. This worked out very well for me, because when I was still overweight, I was usually in a bad mood about it. But, each day the six miles would put me in a better frame of mind. I felt like I was doing something about my weight. The boost in mood also made me more consistent.

Consistency

When you're in a great mood and you're feeling positive and hopeful about life, it's easier to stick to your plan. It also seemed like the act of sticking to the six miles helped me stick to fasting. It was harder to cheat on the plan after putting in such an effort with my steps. I find streaks very motivating, so to have a strong streak of walking going motivated me to keep my streak of sticking to the overall plan going.

Control

I'm a recovering control freak. When I started weighing myself every day in 2015, I quickly realized that I could not control the scale on a day to day basis. This disturbed the control freak within me. I didn't want my whole day to hang on a number that I knew would go up and down rather capriciously. I also knew enough to know that fasting wasn't always going to be 100% within my control due to family events and life in general. Thus, I decided to have a daily goal that was totally in my control: my step goal.

How To Walk 6 Miles A Day

When I formed my plan in January 2016, the moving side of the equation simply stated "walk six miles every day." All I cared about was at the end of the day, my Fitbit had at least 14,000 steps on it, which was six miles for my stride length. I wanted to make this easy on myself, and excuse-proof myself as much as possible. The first way I did this was to tell myself the steps could be as slow as I wanted to go.

Going slow

I knew about myself that in the past "I'm too tired to work out" had been my go to excuse. I had had a Fitbit since December 2014 and would occasionally set step goals for myself, but 2015 was my year of being inconsistent with everything. Despite my inconsistency, I started to recognize that when it came to walking, I always felt like I could walk a few more steps, no matter how tired I was.

In 2016 I told myself that all that was necessary was to walk 6 miles by the end of the day. I would sit down and rest whenever I needed it. There were days where I was getting my 14,000th step just before midnight because I just couldn't seem to fit them in until then. I knew I could never truly use the excuse that I was too tired to take a few more steps. But, there were some excuses I could still use, like "It's too late at night to be outside" or "The weather is too cold/windy/hot/humid." Enter housewalking.

Housewalking

One day, frustrated with myself for being inconsistent with my step goal, I wondered if I could do all of my steps inside. I thought that would be a neat experiment. This meant that I could just walk around my house. I didn't need to wait for my husband to be home so he could watch the kids. I didn't have to drag the kids with me and listen to their complaints of "are we almost done yet?" I simply could walk inside, where, by the way, the climate was always perfectly controlled. I could even walk barefoot, which remains my favorite way to walk. After my first day of successfully walking six miles in my house, I realized I never had an excuse to not get my steps in, barring a major emergency.

Learning How To Like It

Walking sounds so boring. And it can even feel boring at first. When I first got my Fitbit, 10,000 steps felt like such a grind. *Spoiler alert!* Even after years of walking six miles a day, it sometimes still feels like a grind. I keep doing it for the previous reasons I listed above. And I've found there are ways to make walking much more enjoyable.

Music

In the early days, I made myself a playlist of upbeat songs that put me in a good mood. It motivated me to go get my steps in. I even titled the playlist *Get Happy* because that was the whole point: to put myself in a good mood. It had every song I could think of that made me want to dance. There were plenty of guilty pleasure type songs like Carly Rae Jepsen's *Call Me Maybe* and *Walking on Sunshine* by Katrina & The Waves. I'd encourage you to make your own playlist like this. It's amazing how listening to some good music can instantly change your mood. And when you're in a good mood, it's a lot easier to stick to your plan.

Movies and TV
I generally try to limit how much television I watch, so when I do, it feels indulgent. I realized that I could bribe myself to get my steps in by allowing myself to watch Netflix guilt free while I walked. I binge watched shows like *Sherlock* and *Broadchurch*, and it made the miles fly by. And since at the end of it I had walked six miles, I felt accomplished, not guilty.

Podcasts
Eventually I ran out of new shows to watch, and thus began my obsession with podcasts. I found that I had a great opportunity to learn while I was getting my steps in. I fell in love with many different podcasts, such as *Smart Passive Income*, *The Tim Ferriss Show*, Mike Rowe's *The Way I Heard It*, and many many more. The time went by even more quickly than when I was watching TV. And as a bonus, I improved my mind and my body at the same time.

Reconnecting
I also used my walking time to reconnect with people via social media, video messaging, and (my least favorite) telephone calls. I generally felt guilty about being on social media otherwise, but if I was doing something so healthy like walking six miles, the guilt was gone. It also helped me to stay in touch with my out of state family.

How long does it take?
One of the most common questions I get asked is, "How long does it take to walk six miles?" I'm a slow walker. It generally takes me about two solid hours of walking, which is a pace of about three miles per hour. That seems like a big time commitment. But the average American is watching five hours of television per day. When I honestly looked at my day, I realized that I had plenty of time to get my steps in.

Why six miles?

I chose six miles a day rather randomly. I read an article at some point that said a celebrity trainer said moving three miles a day was a guaranteed way to lose weight and keep it off. I figured that I would need more miles since I was such a slow walker. I also figured my metabolism was slower than average, so I doubled the recommendation. I also found the idea of walking six miles a day motivating. I still think of my daily six miles as a true accomplishment each and every day. No matter how crappy or unproductive my day is otherwise, I have at least walked six miles.

Chapter Notes

- The main reason I walk 6 miles a day is that it puts me in a good mood
- Walking six miles a day might not help me lose weight, from a calorie burn perspective.
- Walking was crucial in keeping me busy in my beginning stages of intermittent fasting.
- A daily step goal gave me something I could control, as opposed to the scale, which I cannot control on a day to day basis.
- It's almost impossible for me to be in a bad mood after I've walked six miles.
- Being in a good mood helps me stay consistent with the rest of my plan.
- It helped me to excuse-proof myself: I walked at a slow pace, inside my house.
- Walking can be fun:
    - Watch tv or movies
    - Listen to podcasts
    - Surf social media
    - Talk on the phone
    - Text with friends

CHAPTER 10: ON THE IMPORTANCE OF TRACKING

Without continual growth and progress, such words as improvement, achievement, and success have no meaning. Benjamin Franklin

I believe tracking is the most important part of successfully losing weight and keeping it off for the long term. If you're not tracking your results, it's darn near impossible to see the progress. And you need to be able to see your progress to stick with your plan over the long haul. It helps me that I'm a numbers nerd and I love spreadsheets. But even if you're not a nerd, I encourage you to start tracking. An important part of this journey has been for me to learn how to stop being emotional about my weight. Looking at data takes feelings out of the equation. Is your plan working? The numbers you're tracking will show you in black and white whether it is or not. But first, you have to have a plan.

A Simple, Written Plan

The big difference between 2015 and 2016 for me was that in 2015 I was trying tons of plans, changing things around, and being super emotional and in a hurry. The end of 2015 was when I was starting to feel desperate. I was ready to give up. My weight had plateaued for months. I sat down with my spreadsheet and looked at my notes. I realized I was changing my plan every month, and even then I wasn't sure what my plan was on a week to week basis. I'd quit, start again, change something, and then forget what my plan was, exactly.

In January 2016 I created my plan, wrote it down, and committed to it. It was very important to write the plan down, in detail. I realized that if I didn't know what plan I was doing, the data would not be able to tell me if that plan worked. I have learned that an easy plan is easy to stick to, and a hard plan is hard to stick to. I wanted to be able to stick to my plan for the long term. If you're not sticking to the plan, the data becomes meaningless and tracking pointless. If you find you're not sticking to your plan, the first step is to create a new plan.

What I Track

I track three different numbers: my daily weight, my seven day average, and my steps. I don't count or track calories, macros, or anything else. I have found knowing these three numbers keep me on track for weight loss and maintenance over the long term. I track these numbers whether I'm maintaining or losing. My plan is to track them forever. In the past my pattern has been when I get to my goal weight, I stop tracking. I eventually put the weight back on and then some. I changed that in 2016. Since then, the weight has stayed off, and I've even lost more. For continued success, I continue to track.

Daily Weight

The first thing I do when I wake up in the morning is use the bathroom. The second thing I do is weigh myself. I then log that number in the Fitbit app. I love weighing every single day. In the past, I was terrified of the scale. Weighing every day got me over that fear. It's a daily accountability practice for me: this is where my weight is today. However, I do not care much about this actual number. I have found that my weight fluctuates a lot over the course of a week. In fact, in any given month, it will fluctuate by five or more pounds between my highest and lowest single day weights within a 7 day period. This is enough to make me crazy, which is why I pretty much ignore it. What I'm more interested in is my seven day average weight.

Seven Day Average

I keep track of my running seven day average. I find this by simply adding up my single day weights for the past seven days, and dividing that number by seven. My weight tracking spreadsheet, available for free at https://sixmilestosupper.com/freebies, calculates this for me automatically. The seven day average evens out the peaks and valleys of my daily weight. It helps me to not freak out over a high weight the day after I've had a meal of Chinese food, and to not celebrate too quickly after a single low weight day. It keeps me on an even keel, which is important on a long journey. The seven day average also helps to suss out whether you're in a true plateau, or if the number is just slowly moving down over time.

My Steps

The only thing I care about with my steps is that I have done at least 14,000 by day's end, which is a total of 6 miles. This is a daily goal. I do not allow myself to do 12,000 one day, then make up for it by doing 16,000 the next. It's 14,000 steps every single day, no excuses. For what it's worth, I haven't found an increase in weight loss if I have an increase in steps.

Weighing: Tips For Staying Sane

The scale is a useful servant, and a horrible master. This is a lesson I've had to learn over the course of time. In the beginning of this journey, I'd let a high weight on a single day ruin my whole day. I'd worry and fret over the foods I ate and the exercise I'd done the day before. But I was committed to seeing how this plan would do over the long term, and I learned how to calm down. I started by stepping outside the situation. I was now a scientist performing an experiment. The scale was a data collection tool.

I intentionally changed my reactions to a high weight day. Instead of frustration, I made myself curious. Oh, a high weight today! That's so interesting! I wonder, what made that happen? When I started noticing a pattern of foods that made my weight temporarily increase, I would even eat them again on purpose a week later, to show myself there was no magic. Certain foods make my water weight increase temporarily. The weight comes back off and then some. There's no reason to freak out. I have found it's best to simply log your weight, and watch how your 7 day average is doing over a 2 month period. This helps put things in perspective and puts the focus where it should be: on the big picture.

How Fast Will The Weight Come Off?

Everyone's first question is, how fast will I lose? When I was losing the bulk of my weight (from 207-157) my average was 1.18 pounds per week. When I got into the normal BMI zone, it was much slower: one third of one pound a week, on average. And remember, this is on average. This means that sometimes the weight went up, or I only lost a tiny fraction of a pound. Some lucky souls out there lose more than a pound a week on average. I've met plenty of people who have been very successful with losing the weight and keeping it off, and they averaged about one pound per week. My best advice is to give yourself permission for the weight loss to take a long time. This will eliminate stress and give you the gift of patience. Think in terms of lifetime sustainability and permanent results.

Getting Over The Fear

It was hard to get on the scale that first time. I vividly remember how scared I felt. It takes a whole lot of guts, the first time you do it. It may help to realize that whether you weigh or not, it does not change the reality of your weight being what it is. There's empowerment that comes from getting over a fear. When I finally knew the number, even though it was much higher than I thought it would be, it helped me to make real progress on my journey. If you commit to simply weighing every single day, the fear goes away. Over time, it's no big deal. It's like brushing your teeth, or combing your hair. And while it's true that the number on the scale isn't the only way to measure weight loss success, I've found it's the easiest to be consistent with, and the hardest one to cheat.

Fluctuations

Fluctuations are a reality in my journey. Accepting that fluctuations happen has eliminated a huge amount of stress. Instead of eliminating or fearing the foods that cause the fluctuations, I eat them happily. I prepare myself mentally for the inevitable, but transient, fluctuation that will happen. Sometimes fluctuations happen for no apparent reason at all. Instead of obsessing about the reason, I simply ask myself if I'm being consistent with my plan. If I am, I simply stay the course. Obsessing over reasons why there are fluctuations can lead to stress, which then can lead to inconsistency. It's important to remember that weight loss looks like a heartbeat. The fluctuations go both ways, which is why averaging the numbers can help even out the hills and valleys. It can give you a truer picture of where you're at with your weight.

Water Weight

After literally watching my weight over the course of a few years, I have found that water weight can be deceptive. It's easy to let a high number make you want to swear off a certain kind of food. For example, I have found that peanut butter ramen will routinely spike my weight by 4 or 5 pounds overnight. For a while, this made me scared to eat peanut butter ramen. But, then I started to look at the numbers more closely. I found that when I looked at my daily weights, after 2 or 3 days, my weight was back down to where it was before I ate the ramen, or even lower. It proved to me that it was simply water weight, and that I did not need to fear the temporary rise in weight. Now my strategy is to mentally prepare myself when I am eating a very sugary or salty food. I know that the next day will show an increase, quite possibly a sharp one, but I only need to wait it out. The number will come right back down, and an overall weight loss will eventually happen.

Trends

Even though the seven day average is important to me, the more important thing to me is how my seven day average is trending over the course of two months. I have found that general hormonal fluctuations, water weight fluctuations, and life in general causes any closer examination to be a bit unproductive. The scale moves in its own sweet time. Eventually, it does catch up to my efforts, but sometimes it simply takes a while.

Plateaus

Weight loss plateaus are frustrating. I wish I could tell you I've found a way to prevent them from ever happening. I've talked to lots of people, on many different plans, and my belief is that plateaus are bound to happen. They happen even if you're following your plan 100% to the letter, and you're doing everything right. I believe the key to overcoming a plateau is to be really stubborn, and really patient. It's easier said than done, I know. When you're in the middle of a plateau, you're tempted to change everything. You'll want to exercise more, eat less, and generally make it harder on yourself. I do the opposite.

I have generally found that times of stress are when my weight loss stalls out. I make it a point to relax. I force myself to look at the really big picture. I check in with myself to see if there are any ways I can make my life easier and less stressful. I stay on plan. Since 2016, I have not changed my plan, no matter how stubborn the plateau is. And the plateau has always broken. This is also why I love the seven day average. Sometimes when you look only at the daily weights it can seem to show a plateau, but the seven day average can show that your weight is in reality trending downwards.

Weight Gain

I personally define weight gain as an upward trend of the seven day average, consistently over two months' time. I simply have not experienced weight gain when following this plan consistently. I have had a month or two where I've gained, but this is always due to being off plan for an extended number of days. The scale has never mysteriously started to move up consistently over time. There's always a reason. Checking my consistency and getting back on plan have always been the keys.

Other Ways To Track

After I had my "I've had enough" moment in 2014, I started tracking using three different non-scale methods. I made very little progress that year. I firmly believe that it was because I was afraid of the scale. If I had gotten up the nerve to weigh in 2014, I probably would have had much earlier progress.

Progress Photos
In 2014 I started taking weekly progress photos of myself. If you look at a photo from the beginning of 2014 and the end of 2014, you'll notice that not much changed. That's because progress photos, for me, didn't tell me a whole lot. When I went back and compared photos after I started weighing myself, I realized that even after a 15 pound weight loss, I couldn't tell a difference in the progress photos. Photos just don't provide good data from week to

week. But I continued on with the progress photos, and I'm glad I did. In 2015, I could start to tell more of a difference, and then in 2016 the changes were much more obvious. It is motivating to have accurate photos at every stage of the journey. My recommendation would be, take progress photos, but don't rely on them as your only way of tracking. It's hard to see progress week to week or even month to month. This can lead to frustration, even though in reality your plan might be working.

How clothes fit
This was another method I thought would be helpful, since many websites recommend it as an alternative to weighing. But I found this was a majorly flawed technique in my case. First of all, the clothes I was wearing were way too tight to begin with. I refused to go up to the proper size. And so what would happen was, if I lost weight, the clothes would only feel slightly less tight. Added to this, it's not a very scientific thing. It's more about feeling and guessing. On top of that, if you wear your jeans a few times in a row like I do, you'll trick yourself into thinking the jeans are getting looser. But the minute you wash and dry them, you will realize they're back to fitting like they always have.

Measuring
Measuring, when done properly and consistently can accurately reflect whether a plan is working or not. But the problem is, I found it was too easy to cheat. I could suck in a bit to make myself lose a little bit from week to week. You can also not suck in, but pull the tape a little tighter. Or, you can measure a little higher or a little lower, to get the numbers to be more favorable. When I got honest with myself and stopped sucking it in, I realized I hadn't made any progress at all.

The Importance Of Perspective

You'll notice that my tracking focuses on the long view. I find it's a waste of energy to get worked up on daily or even weekly fluctuations in weight. Switching my focus on the long term helped me relax and have patience in 2016. When I set a goal of 1 pound a week, and even accepted a half a pound a week as a victory, I was able to focus on the long view. To take it even further, what's truly important to me is, am I doing the things that will make it so that five years from now I am going to be at a healthy weight? It puts a bad day, or even a bad week into perspective. It meant thinking in terms of years, and lifelong sustainability. I believe this was crucial to losing the weight and maintaining the weight loss over time.

Chapter Notes

- Tracking is critical to my weight loss and maintenance success
- Tracking is a surefire way to know if your plan is working. It takes feelings out of the equation
- Daily weighing keeps me accountable
- The running 7 day average keeps me sane
- Fluctuations and plateaus happen, and it's best not to freak out and change your plan because of them
- Reasons plateaus happen: inconsistency, stress, and no good reason at all
- The most important thing I watch is the trend. How is the weight trending over 2 months time?

CHAPTER 11: INTERMITTENT FASTING AND PERIODS

Women complain about premenstrual syndrome, but I think of it as the only time of the month that I can be myself. -Roseanne Barr

One fear I had when I was starting intermittent fasting was that it would screw up my hormones. I really hated the idea of my period going all wonky, and this was yet another reason why I pushed my window out very slowly. As it turns out, my periods were never affected by intermittent fasting. I compiled all the data of my periods since starting intermittent fasting, and found that my period stayed just as regular, if not more so, than when I was overweight and eating normally. I still get crampy and bloated and moody. But that's not to say that no more can be said on the subject; I found that my period affected my intermittent fasting.

Period Hunger

As I discussed earlier, I have found that around that time of the month, I experience a sharp increase in hunger in my fasting window. This generally happens a few days before my period starts. In the beginning I found that it was helpful to simply open my eating window earlier, or eat my OMAD a bit earlier in the day. I always listened to my body, and never beat myself up if I needed the meal to be earlier. As time went on, probably because I was simply a more experienced faster, I found that I didn't need to make those adjustments.

Bad Mood

I recognized, thanks in part to my husband, that there was one day in particular, just before my period, where my mood changed rather drastically. I do not think this was directly related to intermittent fasting, per se. I think I was simply paying more attention to how I was feeling, and checking in with myself more often, and I discovered this pattern. My husband started to bring me "emergency chocolate" for these times. This generally looked like one day out of the month, wherein I would have an afternoon snack of chocolate. Again, no guilt allowed. And you know what? It put me in a better mood.

Increased Appetite

I have also noticed that during my period, I have a larger appetite at my meal. I tend to eat more servings and bigger portions. I simply obey my hunger and eat until I'm good and full. I find that I do not feel miserable afterwards. When I first noticed this pattern, I was worried that I would gain weight. Now I recognize it as a transient phase, and that my appetite will return to normal when the period is over.

Increased Need For Sleep

Although I am generally an early riser and I don't generally require more than 6 hours of sleep, this changes during my period. I find I need a couple more hours of sleep each night, and I simply allow myself to take the extra rest. I have found I feel much better, and function at a higher level if I simply allow myself to sleep more during that time of the month. I don't allow myself to feel guilty for sleeping more.

Slower Walking Speed

I already walk at a pretty slow pace, but there's something about my period that makes me feel more tired. And when I'm feeling tired, I want to walk slower. So I do. Sometimes it's more of a saunter than it is a walk, but going slower allows me to enjoy it. I've tried pushing myself to walk faster than I feel like I want to, but I find it makes me miserable. And the last thing I want to do during my period is feel more miserable. Since I allow myself to just do my steps slowly, I stay consistent with getting them in. This gives me a win for the day. I have found that it improves my mood vastly. And staying in as good a mood as possible is key for me staying on the rest of the plan.

Weight Fluctuations

Life's not fair. Just at the moment you're feeling the most vulnerable, the moodiest, and the crampiest, the scale will start to fluctuate like mad. I have found that my weight shifts constantly and illogically all throughout my period. Some months the numbers are consistently higher. Some months I'll have high days and low days mixed throughout the duration. I continue to weigh every day and I continue to stick to my plan, but I have learned to ignore the numbers from this week. Because it can be comical how the numbers go up and down, I almost look forward to my period week. Almost.

Chapter Notes

- I learned to listen to my body and open my eating window early if necessary.
- Emergency chocolate was a helpful crutch to get me through PMS.
- I require more food and sleep during my period.
- I need to walk slower.

- The scale will be ridiculous.
    - I will continue to weigh every day
    - I will continue to stick to my plan
    - I will basically ignore the numbers from this week

CHAPTER 12: INTERMITTENT FASTING AND EMOTIONAL EATING

I use food for the same reasons an addict uses drugs: to comfort, to soothe to ease stress. - Oprah Winfrey

Perhaps the most valuable thing I've gotten out of intermittent fasting, even more valuable than the weight loss itself, has been how intermittent fasting has freed me from emotional eating. I never realized, before intermittent fasting, how often I was eating for reasons other than true hunger. I ate because I was stressed, tired, lonely, and bored. Eating had also become the most exciting part of my day; ironic, since it was also the most stressful. Intermittent fasting helped me learn how to eat appropriately.

No Forbidden Foods

I used to think certain foods were forbidden, that I was being "bad" if I ate them. Before intermittent fasting, eating a chocolate chip cookie was not a simple act. I would eat the cookie. *That cookie was delicious!* Eating the cookie made me feel good. But then I would immediately feel guilty. *How dare you eat the cookie! You're so overweight!* Then I would eat another cookie to make myself feel better. I would enjoy the taste for a moment, but then I felt more guilt. The rebellious side of me would overindulge just to try to prove some ridiculous point. In fact, this drama didn't just play out in my head when I was eating cookies. It happened at pretty much every meal, and it was exhausting. My experience with intermittent fasting has helped heal my relationship with food.

January 2016 is when I officially told myself there are no forbidden foods. My idea was that all foods were allowed during my eating window. There was to be no guilt for whatever I ate during the eating window. As long as I was obeying the rule of fasting during fasting time, and eating during eating time, I was on plan. This seemed like an insane plan at first. I figured it would mean that I would binge endlessly on junk food during my eating window. Instead, I found that over time, my cravings for my previously forbidden foods lessened. And when I did eat those foods, I found that I had stopping power.

Forbidden fruit tastes the sweetest. How true I found that to be! All the things that seemed so seductive when I wasn't allowed to have them, didn't seem as tempting when they were completely allowed. It's taken time, of course. In the beginning I ate more donuts and sweets in my eating window. The first surprising thing I found was that when I allowed myself to eat however many I wanted, guilt free, I simply didn't eat as many as I would have previously, when I was trying to "be good."

And I think that's an important point here. My tactic here was not to eat sweets in moderation. My whole life I've been attempting moderation, and it frequently made me overindulge. Instead, I honestly allow myself to eat as much as I want. It took the emotion out of it for me, and gave me the ability to enjoy the foods fully. This gave me the ability to focus on whether or not I was truly satisfied.

Eating My Emotions

As it turns out, when I was overweight, I also ate for many reasons other than hunger. I had no idea I was doing this until I started intermittent fasting. When I was overweight, I honestly thought I was only eating when I was hungry. And to an extent, that was true. Every time I ate, it was because I *felt* hungry. It was only when I was fasting that I realized many different emotions made me feel hungry, but it wasn't true hunger.

Normally, I found fasting relatively easy when I was being consistent with it. My body would only feel hungry during the eating window. But occasionally I'd start to feel a sudden hunger out of the blue during my fasting window. Caving into the hunger wasn't an option for me, so I had to figure out another way to handle it. I usually just kept myself busy and found that it would go away on its own. Eventually I started to see a pattern. I was getting hungry every time I was stressed.

My husband was a Realtor at the time, and our income was variable. We were never sure if a deal would actually close or not, and this was a major stress in my life. Sure enough, every time there was a budget meeting, or some issue popped up with a deal that was under contract, I felt incredibly hungry. I realized I had to figure out other ways to cope with stress. I found talking out my feelings with my husband, going for walks, and journaling all helped me greatly. Ultimately, I started actively eliminating stress from my life by taking action on the things that were stressing me out.

It's A Process

Learning how to deal with emotional eating took a long time. I still consider myself a work in progress. I am aware that I have a natural tendency to emotionally eat, and I'm well aware that it is a habit that can creep back in at any time. To prevent this, I constantly check in with myself at each meal while I'm eating. If I find myself feeling stressed while I am eating, I remind myself to slow down and enjoy my meal. I consciously make myself relax. I pay close attention to whether I'm feeling full or not. And most importantly, I am intentional about taking action on the thing that was stressing me out in the first place. I've been relieved to find that even on cheat day, I am not eating emotionally. It's a process that has taken patience and effort over time.

Chapter Notes

- I never understood how much I was emotionally eating until I started intermittent fasting
- Being consistent with intermittent fasting requires that you handle stress and other emotions in ways other than eating
- Alternatives to emotional eating that I found helpful:
    - Going for a walk
    - Journaling
    - Talking it out
    - Taking a nap
    - Taking action on whatever was stressing me out
- Getting rid of the idea of forbidden foods helped me to gain control over my emotional eating
    - I do not allow myself to feel guilty for eating any foods I eat
    - Focusing on moderation generally made me feel deprived and led to overindulging
    - I now have excellent stopping power
    - Overall, I crave less of those previously forbidden foods

CHAPTER 13: THE IMPORTANCE OF MINDSET

The passion for stretching yourself and sticking to it, even (or especially) when it's not going well, is the hallmark of the growth mindset. This is the mindset that allows people to thrive during some of the most challenging times in their lives. -Carol S. Dweck, Mindset: The New Psychology Of Success

One of the best things I did for myself in 2014 was to start to read books about self-improvement and mindset. My husband had just started a career in real estate, and he was constantly reading books by authors like Zig Ziglar, Brian Tracy, and Darren Hardy. I found that reading these types of books helped me to discover some things about myself that surprised me. Previously, I thought I was a positive person overall, with a great mindset. As it turned out, I had a lot of work to do in this department.

Changing Negative Self-Talk

The biggest revelation I had was that my self-talk was incredibly negative. Your self-talk, also known as your inner dialogue, is the constant conversation that's going on in your head. It's the story you're telling yourself about yourself. When I started noticing what I was saying about myself, it was quite shocking. I would routinely call myself fat, dumb, and a failure. These are things I would never say to another human being. But with myself, I had no filter, and almost no boundaries on the negativity I could pour on myself.

Over time, I found that I was able to change my negative self talk. I'm still very much a work in progress, but I have made major improvements. The act of recognizing I was talking negatively to myself was half the battle. The other half of the battle was catching myself and changing my self-talk to something more honest and positive. I found that sometimes there was an underlying truth to the negativity, so it wasn't enough to only tell myself not to say that about myself. Example:

Negative self-talk: Gosh, Kayla, you're so fat.
Reality at the time: I was 45 pounds overweight.
Self-correction in my head: I'm currently 45 pounds overweight. I am making progress towards a healthy weight by practicing intermittent fasting and walking 6 miles a day.

I also liked to take it a step further than the correction. Every time I caught myself saying mean things to myself, I'd make myself come up with 5 or 10 nice compliments to pay myself. My negative talk was almost constant at first. Over time, it became less frequent, and at this time it is quite rare for me to experience it. Changing my self-talk put me in a more positive mood, which then made me a better mother and wife, and gave me a happier life overall.

Limiting Beliefs

I read Tony Robbins' book *Awaken the Giant Within*, and it educated me about the idea of limiting beliefs. This concept is intertwined with your self-talk. Your limiting beliefs are the beliefs that you've adopted about yourself which can hold you back. One limiting belief I had was that I had a bad metabolism. I believed that I was doomed to struggle with my weight. One example that Tony gave in his book, which still stands out in my mind years later, is about homelessness. He has worked extensively with the homeless, and he has found that those people who identify as homeless tend to stay homeless, but those who identify as people who are temporarily without a home tend to get back on their feet. The idea is, our limiting beliefs prevent us from taking action, because we believe those are things about our lives we cannot change. If you think a situation is permanent, you do not try to change it. I started telling myself that my metabolism was fine, and that I was a person who was temporarily overweight. This led me to continue taking action to lose the weight, even when I had setbacks.

Impostor Syndrome

This is something I had to deal with as I started to lose weight. Impostor syndrome is when a person doubts their own accomplishments and fears they'll be exposed as a fraud. I felt this way about weight loss. I was afraid that after I lost weight, people would think of me as a fat person who was just trying to be skinny. Yes, that might sound totally irrational, but it was something I had to figure out. I actually got a handle on impostor syndrome after I learned about spotlight syndrome.

Spotlight Syndrome

Most people believe everyone in the room is focused on them. The truth is, no one is paying that much attention to you or me. Most people are concerned with their own selves. I eventually started to realize that people in general aren't really thinking about me. They have their own lives to focus on.

Ironically, I found this truth out when I was getting upset with people for not noticing my weight loss. Before this I thought everyone was focused on me, and that they were obsessed with my weight. When no one said anything after I lost 15 or 20 pounds, I started to realize I was suffering from spotlight syndrome. As it turns out, we are actually all pretty self-absorbed.

A quote I heard that helped me was: your best friend in the whole world thinks more about a hangnail he has, than he thinks about a major problem you're having in your own life. When I thought about this, I realized that it was true. I analyzed how often I thought of my own problems and myself throughout the course of the day. I thought of myself constantly. On the other hand, how often had I thought of my close family member who was dealing with a terrible disease? On a good day, it crossed my mind once.

This seems depressing, on the face of it. However, I have found it incredibly freeing. It's led to me taking the road less traveled in many areas of my life, and it's made me less nervous in social situations. Instead of being worried about other people's opinions, I focus on whether a particular decision is right for me personally. This also helped me conquer impostor syndrome. People simply aren't putting that much thought into my weight or my decisions. My weight loss is at best a passing thought in their life.

Murdering Perfectionism

I used to think of perfectionism as a personality trait to be proud of. It made me a high achiever, and I always strived to be excellent at everything I tried. But perfectionism has a dark side. First of all, it made me miserable. If I started pursuing an interest like computer programming, I enjoyed it at first. But as soon as it stopped coming easy, I quit. I was terrified of looking incompetent. I never wanted to look like a failure. My perfectionist tendencies led me to have a fixed mindset, which Carol Dweck discusses at length in her excellent book, *Mindset*. I fortunately found and read that book in 2016, and it helped me to change to a growth mindset.

A fixed mindset makes weight loss difficult. It's what would make me completely quit on a plan the first time I messed up. It was all or nothing. It was either perfect eating on the diet or no plan at all. Learning to tame my perfectionism took time. I credit my cheat days for helping me to understand that being a B+ student has its perks. It's a much more relaxed way to live. I found I could easily get back on plan when I went off, because I was no longer under the illusion that I was perfect.

Taking Care Of Myself

Learning how to simply be nicer to myself has been quite a process. It sounds trivial, but it's not. If you're allowing negative self-talk, you're constantly being mean to yourself, which can make your days miserable. Changing my self-talk was an important aspect of being nicer to myself, but it wasn't the only thing.

Checking In
It's been enormously helpful to learn how to check in with myself. For example, in the past, if I overate at a meal, I would beat myself up and feel guilty that I'd overdone it. During this journey, I stopped beating myself up and started checking in instead. Here's how that looks for me now. Let's say I overeat at a meal. I do not browbeat myself. I simply ask myself how I am feeling. Am I stressed about something right now? If I am stressed, I make it a point to take action on whatever it is that is stressing me out. If I'm not stressed, I ask if I'm tired. If I'm tired, I give myself a guilt-free nap, or get in the bed earlier that night. It has been a process of learning why I am doing the things I am doing, and then taking positive actions to improve my behavior for the future.

Me Time
I have found that the more I take care of myself, and the nicer I am to myself, the easier the weight loss journey has become. An important thing for me was giving myself "Me Time." I know, it sounds selfish at first. But I have found that if I give myself 30 minutes each day, to simply be by myself, or to relax with a book, or to go for a walk, I feel rejuvenated. I end up being a better mother, wife, and person in general.

Slow And Steady

One major mindset shift that happened in 2016 was from demanding fast results of myself, to accepting slow and steady results. I gave myself permission for my weight loss journey to take a long time. By this time I realized that no one was paying attention to my weight loss anyway. I had put loads of pressure on myself in 2015 to get all the weight off fast, which led to lots of stress. I heard a great quote from Jocko Willink that the Navy SEALs use: slow is smooth, and smooth is fast. The general idea is that when we rush, we make mistakes, and when we make mistakes, the thing we're doing takes longer. Instead, we should focus on going slow and staying the course. This was one of my most important mindset shifts.

Chapter Notes

- Proper mindset is crucially important to weight loss
- Find out what your self-limiting beliefs are and deal with them
- Impostor syndrome can sabotage your success. You might feel like you're a fraud if you lose weight, but this is all in your head.
- Spotlight syndrome tricks us into thinking that everyone is watching every move we make, when in reality everyone's pretty self-absorbed
- Murdering perfectionism helps you get back on plan after you get off
- Being nicer to yourself is critically important to long-term success. Negative self-talk sabotages your efforts over the long haul.

CHAPTER 14: HOW TO STAY MOTIVATED

Wanting something is not enough. You must hunger for it. Your motivation must be absolutely compelling in order to overcome the obstacles that will invariably come your way. -Les Brown

The weight loss journey is long. Even if you have 50 pounds to lose, and you lose at the rate of one pound a week, that still means sticking with your plan consistently for an entire year. I can almost guarantee you that there will be times when you'll lose motivation. I found that stress, hormones, and life in general would occasionally trip me up and make me consider quitting or changing my plan. It was important to learn how to stay motivated. Motivation is tricky because different tactics work for different people.

Finding Your Why

Figuring out the why behind weight loss can help you stay motivated for the long term. It's not enough to say "I want to lose weight." You need to ask yourself why. And the deeper you can go with this, the better off you're going to be. The Toyota Motor Corporation has done this for years to thoroughly troubleshoot and get to the root cause of a problem. At each answer, they again ask why. Try doing it 5 times for any goal you're wanting to achieve, and you'll find much deeper motivation. Some of the deeper whys for my weight loss were:
- I want to be able to keep up with my kids
- I want to live life fully and not feel held back because of my

weight
- I want to feel confident when I'm around other people

Finding the why behind your goals is important. But it's also important to motivate yourself in other ways. And that takes some self-exploration.

What Makes You Tick?

The real key is to figure out what makes you tick. You need to start asking yourself what lights a fire under you. You might find you don't really know what makes you tick when it comes to weight loss. I certainly felt that way in the beginning. It helps to look at areas of your life where you are already getting stuff done. For example, if you keep a really clean house, how do you do that? Or if you successfully got out of debt, what helped you achieve that goal? Was it treating yourself to a luxurious vacation? Buying yourself something? Was it a countdown to a date? A checklist? Whatever it was, try to adopt those same techniques and apply them to your weight loss goals.

What Worked For Me

In 2011-2012 we paid off a large amount of debt. I looked at what motivated me during that time, and one thing that stood out was that I kept track of how the number was coming down over time. I then transferred that technique over to weight loss by tracking my weight over time in a spreadsheet. I was able to watch how my weight was coming down over time, and it kept me motivated.

For me, the most motivational thing is to be able to see that I am making progress, especially if that is in the form of a list. Yes, I know that sounds weird and boring to some of you. But some of you get it. Having a to do list helps me get stuff done. So in 2016 I made myself a weight loss checklist that looked like this:

Get down to a 7 day average of 200 (should hit by February 5)

Get down to a 7 day average of 195 (should hit by March 11)

Get down to a 7 day average of 190 (should hit by April 15)

I did this in five pound increments all the way down to my goal weight. The date goal in parentheses was to remind me of about how long it would take, based on my one pound per week goal. As I hit the goals, it looked like this:

~~Get down to a 7 day average of 200 (should hit by February 5)~~
Achieved on January 26

~~Get down to a 7 day average of 195 (should hit by March 11)~~
Achieved on March 3

~~Get down to a 7 day average of 190 (should hit by April 15)~~
Achieved on April 6

I could see the proof in black and white: I was making progress. I would hit my goals eventually. Breaking my big goal into small, manageable subgoals made the whole thing seem less overwhelming. And in my head, I even went further: I was only focused on the next pound of weight loss. When I was at 198, I was just focused on seeing a 197 show up on the scale. It almost became a little game to me.

The Power Of Personal Bests

I had found setting personal bests motivated me in 2015 when I started powerlifting. It showed me that I was getting better each week. In 2016 I decided to incorporate personal bests into my walking. I set goals for personal bests for steps each month. I ended up getting over 40,000 steps in a single day by October. This also made my daily goal of 14,000 steps seem easy by comparison. I found that doing something hard one day out of the month was enough. My daily plan felt almost effortless, and the once a month challenge helped me to grow and be mentally tougher. This mental toughness helped me to stay on plan and not give up when the scale was moving slower than I hoped it would.

What Doesn't Work?

There were things I tried to motivate myself that didn't work for me. For example, telling myself I'd buy myself something at a certain weight loss milestone was a bad idea. Why? First of all, things don't tend to excite me. I hate shopping, and I don't like having a lot of stuff. Secondly, what usually happened was that when I hit the milestone, for example, 15 pounds lost, we'd be tight on money. So then I couldn't buy myself those cool wireless headphones, and I felt frustrated rather than motivated.

Goal pants were not very motivating either. The reason for this was that it was too vague. I had some goal pants, and there was a long stretch of time from when I could get them on and zipped up until I could actually fit into them well enough to want to wear them out in public. And even then, they were slightly uncomfortable. Basically, it was hard to know when I had truly achieved the goal of "Fit into goal jeans."

Food Rewards?
One thing I never did, and I still refuse to do, is reward myself with food. My plan, after all, allows me to eat all the foods that I want, every day. On top of that, I give myself a cheat day every week. There were times during the journey that I would recognize a temptation to reward myself with food. For example, I would think of rewarding myself with a pint of Ben and Jerry's when I lost 30 pounds. I saw that as a red flag: it meant I was still considering certain foods forbidden. I then intentionally made it a point to get some of that kind of food right away and either eat it in my regular eating window, or on cheat day. I worked very hard to eliminate the notion from my mind that any foods were forbidden, and it's one of the best things that has come out of this entire journey.

Motivation

Weight loss, it should be noted, becomes its own reward. I found the more I lost, the less I needed other forms of motivation. It's another unfair reality about weight loss: you need motivation in the beginning, and that's when it's hardest to motivate yourself. When you start to be successful at it, you need the motivation less, but that's when motivation is the easiest to access.

Chapter Notes

- There is no one best method for motivating yourself
- Occasional challenges that feel tough can help you become mentally stronger, such as setting a personal best
- Find other areas in your life where you have been successful and apply those techniques to your weight loss
- Figuring out what makes you tick will help you find the right ways to motivate yourself
- What worked for me:
    - A checklist broken down into 5 pound increments
    - Setting personal bests
    - Weight loss also became its own reward
- What didn't work for me:
    - Physical rewards - I'm not motivated by material goods
    - Goal pants - it was too hard to tell when I'd achieved that goal
- I never reward myself with food. In my plan no foods are forbidden, so I eat them whenever I want

CHAPTER 15: HOW TO MAINTAIN

Success is a journey. Not a destination. -Arthur Ashe

Weight loss maintenance was always a mystery to me. In the past when I reached my goal weight, I didn't know what to do. I assumed that I could start eating like a normal person. And eventually, the weight would return with a vengeance. In 2014, I was determined to figure out this piece of the puzzle, because weight loss success seemed pointless without it.

With intermittent fasting in particular, I wasn't really sure how this would look. Would I always need to practice intermittent fasting? Could I go back to three meals a day? How strict would I need to be? How hard was it going to be to maintain my loss? In November 2016 until September 2017, I embarked on finding those answers.

I stayed in the experimental mindset when I went into maintenance mode. I again borrowed a hack from Tim Ferriss: always search for the Minimum Effective Dose. The idea was, what's the most laid back I can be with this plan, but still keep the weight off? I realized that if I went back to eating how I ate when I was 222 pounds, I would eventually go back to weighing 222. I knew my eating would need to look different than it did at 222. The key was figuring out the balance. What worked for me was to continue to have a plan, continue to track, and give myself a five pound leeway.

Have A Plan

My plan was to experiment with various eating plans. I sometimes ate three times a day, usually twice, sometimes once. I wanted to see how loosey goosey I could be, while still not gaining weight. I didn't keep very accurate notes of what I was doing during this time, though I wish I would have. My goal was to be very relaxed, and see if the weight came back or not. Generally speaking, I was eating either lunch and supper, or supper and late night snacks with my husband. I was surprised to find that even though I was giving myself permission to eat however I wanted, I found that overall I preferred intermittent fasting.

I felt better with intermittent fasting, and I also found I was more productive as well. I enjoy the time savings, and the not having to think about food for a large part of the day. I enjoyed having supper and then late night snacks with my husband, which felt completely luxurious to me. Enjoyment of your plan is important. If you don't enjoy what you're doing, eventually you'll stop doing it.

Continue To Track

The most important thing I did was to continue to track my weight by weighing every day. It was still the same routine: wake up, use the bathroom, then get on the scale. Log the weight in my Fitbit app. Every Friday, I input those numbers into my spreadsheet to keep track of my seven day average. I was not concerned with the number fluctuating higher or lower. I concentrated on not letting my seven day average go too high. I think everyone's going to have a different comfort zone here, but mine was 5 pounds from where I entered maintenance mode.

I have personally decided to weigh every day for the rest of my life. When I look back to those times where I lost weight, but I did not keep it off, a common thread was that I stopped weighing myself. If I weigh every day, I'll always know exactly right where I'm at, which is empowering. It helps to think of it as just another daily task like brushing my teeth or balancing my checkbook.

A 5 Pound Leeway

I gave myself a five pound leeway, meaning that I didn't feel the need to try to intentionally lose weight until my seven day average consistently went above five pounds over the weight I entered maintenance mode at. Why five pounds? It's completely arbitrary. When I looked back at my seven day average, I realized that it didn't vary easily, but it did vary some. I figured that if I only gave myself two or three pounds, I'd be constantly stressing out over normal weight fluctuations.

I wanted to have as much freedom as possible. On the other hand, the thought of giving myself ten pounds of leeway felt like too much. I thought it'd feel a bit overwhelming to let the weight get that far up before I did something about it. So, I settled on five. I found that I could be very loose with my plan and still maintain within that range with what felt like almost no effort at all. My old patterns of stress eating did not come back, I think because I had finally learned to tell stress hunger from true hunger, and I'd also found better ways to cope with the stress.

Chapter Notes

- Remember that if you go back to eating how you used to eat, you will go back to weighing what you used to weigh
- Have a plan that feels easy
- Continue to track
- Give yourself some leeway. I like 5 pounds.

EPILOGUE

Action cures fear. -David J. Schwartz

Weight Loss: Is It Worth It?

Weight loss success can almost be as scary as failure. I had lots of fears about being successful with weight loss. What if I lost the weight, but then gained it all back? What if I looked worse after I lost weight? What if my friends no longer liked me? What if I changed into a jerk, because I was skinny? What if my husband liked me less when I lost weight? What if it hurt our marriage? I am thrilled that I was able to push past these fears, because as it turns out, they were completely unfounded.

I found that weight loss changed my life for the better. I had tons more energy. I felt more positive and confident about life. This led me to be a better mother and wife, because I felt better. I also started living life more fully, because I wasn't letting insecurities hold me back from trying new experiences. I started putting myself out there more. As it turns out, when I was overweight, I tended to be more judgmental and harsh than when I got down to a normal weight. I started going from a fixed mindset to a growth mindset. Instead of being threatened by other people's success, I was encouraged by it.

Starting my Youtube channel, *Six Miles To Supper,* in 2017 was a huge step for my personal growth. In the past I was terrified of putting myself out there in that way, especially making my weight public. I was afraid that by posting videos about weight loss, I'd have to endure a constant barrage of negativity and criticism. Instead I found that there were lots of people who resonated with what I was saying. I've received more encouragement than I could have ever imagined. In August 2018 I walked 100,000 steps (43.2 miles) in a single day, and with the help of my audience raised over $10,000 to dig a well in Jezza, Uganda for widows and orphans, through my favorite charity, Kinship United.

The confidence I gained through losing the weight and keeping it off, along with my newfound knowledge of spotlight syndrome gave me the courage to try an entirely new and adventurous lifestyle: full-time RVing across the country with my husband and three kids. I've traveled more in the past six months since starting this adventure than I have for the past 14 years. When I was overweight, I kept putting off life. Now I'm grabbing it by the horns.

There were times in this journey, particularly by the beginning of 2016, when I was almost ready to give up. By the grace of God, I didn't. I kept being stubborn, kept getting back on track when I lost my way, and eventually I found success. It was not always easy, and in fact, sometimes it felt really hard. There were times when I was getting my 14,000th step right before the stroke of midnight. There were other times when I wanted to stuff my face instead of talk out what was really bothering me. But with each challenge, I gained new strength, and I improved my life. Looking back over this journey, I can say without reservation, it has been so worth it.

ABOUT THE AUTHOR

Kayla Cox

When she's not homeschooling her three kids, running the day to day operations of her household, or hanging out with her amazing husband, Kayla spends her time reading and writing and making videos. She walks six miles a day and loves exploring God's green earth every chance she gets. You can find more intermittent fasting resources on her website sixmilestosupper.com or on her Youtube channel, Six Miles To Supper.

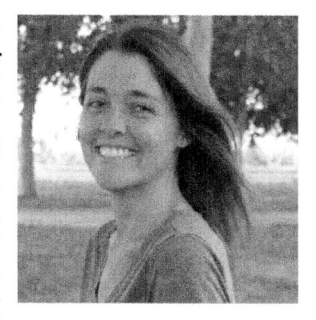

BOOKS BY THIS AUTHOR

Overcoming Weight Loss Obstacles: How To Keep Going When Things Get Difficult

Frustrating obstacles appear in every weight loss journey. Plateaus, overeating, slow weight loss, emotional eating, and weight gain are a few of the common roadblocks that can cause you to quit before you hit your goal weight. The good news is, all these obstacles can be overcome. Each chapter in this book will mentally prepare you for the challenges you are likely to face and will give you tips on how to overcome each one. It will help you to focus on the why behind losing weight and on the big picture, so that you continue to make progress in a sustainable way.

Printed in Great Britain
by Amazon